CLINICIAN'S DESK REFERENCE

Parkinson's Disease

Donald G Grosset

Katherine A Grosset

Institute of Neurological Sciences,
Southern General Hospital,
Glasgow, UK

Michael S Okun

Hubert H Fernandez

Movement Disorders Center,
McKnight Brain Institute,
University of Florida,
Gainesville, Florida, USA

MANSON PUBLISHING

ISBN: 978-1-84076-101-6

For full details of all Manson Publishing titles please write to:
Manson Publishing Ltd, 73 Corringham Road, London NW11 7DL, UK.
Tel: +44(0)20 8905 5150
Fax: +44(0)20 8201 9233
Website: www.mansonpublishing.com

Commissioning editor: Jill Northcott
Project manager, book and diagram design: Ayala Kingsley
Copy editor: Joanna Brocklesby
Indexer: Jill Dormon
Illustrations: DiacriTech
Colour reproduction: Tenon & Polert Colour Scanning Ltd, Hong Kong
Printed by: Grafos SA, Barcelona, Spain

Contents

Contributors

Chapters 1, 2, 3, 4

Donald G. Grosset, BSc MBChB MD FRCP
Consultant Neurologist
Katherine A. Grosset, MBChB MRCGP(1989) MD
Hospital Practitioner

Institute of Neurological Sciences,
Southern General Hospital,
Glasgow, UK

Chapters 4, 5, 7

Hubert H. Fernandez, MD
Michael S. Okun, MD
Co-Directors

Movement Disorders Center,
McKnight Brain Institute, University of Florida,
Gainesville, Florida, USA

Chapter 6

Maria L. Moro-de-Casillas, MD
Movement Disorders Fellow
Joseph H. Friedman, MD
Clinical Professor
Kelvin L. Chou, MD
Clinical Assistant Professor

Department of Clinical Neurosciences, Brown Medical
School,
NeuroHealth Parkinson's Disease and Movement
Disorders Center,
Warwick, Rhode Island, USA

Melissa Amick, PhD
Research Associate

Department of Psychiatry and Human Behavior,
Brown Medical School,
Staff Neuropsychologist, Department of Rehabilitation
Medicine,
Memorial Hospital of Rhode Island,
Pawtucket, Rhode Island, USA

Chapter 8

Janet Romrell, PA-C
Physician Assistant

Movement Disorders Center,
University of Florida,
Gainesville, Florida, USA

Chapter 9

Keith J. Myers, MBA, PT
Portia Gardner-Smith, OTR/L, CHT

Shands Healthcare,
Department of Rehabilitation Services, University of
Florida
Gainesville, Florida, USA

Chapter 10

John C. Rosenbek, PhD
Harrison N. Jones, MA

Department of Communicative Disorders, University of
Florida
Gainesville, Florida, USA

Chapter 11

Kathrynne Holden, MS, RD
President

Five Star Living, Inc.
Springfield, Missouri, USA

Chapter 12

Theresa A. McClain, MSN, ARNP
Robert A. Hauser, MD, MBA

Department of Neurology
Parkinson's Disease and Movement Disorders Center
University of South Florida,
Tampa, Florida, USA

Acknowledgements

The authors would like to gratefully acknowledge the
following people for their kind and expert assistance in
the preparation of this book: the authors of the individual chapters; the University of Florida's Greg Crucian for
his assistance with Chapter 10; those who assisted with
illustrations – Angela O'Donnell, Dr Edward Newman,
Dr Jim Patterson, Atchar Sudhyadhom, Elaine Tyrrell,
Dr Jerry Vitek, Dr Benjamin Walter, Dr Ludvic Zrinzo,
and for secretarial assistance – Margaret Crawford and
Elizabeth Jackson.

Introduction

WE HAVE TRIED, in writing this book, to take a unique approach to Parkinson's disease and one that we hope will provide a concise, practical and useful resource for the reader. The book adopts a 'key facts' method of explaining the disease, its diagnosis, differentiation from other conditions, assessment, and treatment. The chapters are laid out in an easy-to-read style, with bulleted points throughout and a wealth of helpful diagrams and photographs.

The management of motor symptoms in relation to drug treatment, from initial presentation through the period of fluctuating disease to complex advanced stages, is reviewed, but there is also specific attention paid to the non-motor aspects, which have come under closer scrutiny in recent years. We have also included a complete section on surgical therapies. Moreover, the non-pharmacological management of Parkinson's disease is also specifically addressed, with sections regarding the input from multidisciplinary, allied team professionals, including physiotherapy, occupational therapy, speech and language, dietetics, and complementary therapy. We also did not want to forget the important and influential role of the Parkinson's disease nurse specialist who is often a key point of coordination of services for patients, including the medical and allied professionals, and wider aspects of social care and involvement and informing of the patient's carers and family. We provide a detailed glossary of terms used in this field, and a summary of key resources, in particular the patient representative bodies and self-help organizations which provide so much assistance to patients and their carers, as well as support for research.

In Chapter 1, *Parkinson's disease facts and figures*, we offer a logical sequence moving from incidence and prevalence figures and survival data, through to the causes and risk factors associated with the condition, and then on to the genetic and environmental ones. In this chapter we also address rates of progression of Parkinson's disease, a frequent question by patients and their carers. The reader will find clear summary statements, essentially a 'mini evidence-based summary' on this and many points. And where data are controversial or contradictory, we similarly highlight these key points. Lastly, the pathophysiology and neuropathology of Parkinson's are considered, with a review of mitochondrial dysfunction and oxidative stress.

In Chapter 2, *Clinical diagnosis of parkinsonism and tremor*, we look at diagnostic issues, first by examining the question of when symptoms develop, then by describing the cardinal features of the disease and their clinical tests, and finally the additional or supporting features are reviewed. There is then a consideration of problems relating to diagnosis, measured against the various diagnostic clinical criteria that have been proposed for PD. Conditions which are sometimes confused in clinical practice with Parkinson's disease are outlined, together with a summary of the 'red flags' – a key guide to recognizing what is and is not PD.

In Chapter 3, *Diagnostic testing and neuroimaging*, the role of these techniques is summarized. While clinical diagnosis remains the main approach for this condition, there are situations where diagnostic tests need to be performed. The use of antiparkinson therapy is itself sometimes an investigative test (a 'trial of therapy') to support a possible PD diagnosis. There are also the more recent developments; testing the sense of smell – which is impaired in Parkinson's disease and is usually normal in other movement disorders – and the use of functional dopaminergic imaging. In this latter category the two main types of imaging with PET and SPECT scans are examined. While structural imaging does not have a major role in the diagnosis of Parkinson's disease, the reasons why it should be used in some cases, and the type of findings which may be seen, are also covered.

In Chapter 4, *Drug treatment of Parkinson's disease*, the treatment of both motor and non-motor features is reviewed in detail, with consideration of current anti-PD drugs under their respective classes.

The non-motor features are given their own section (Chapter 5, *Nonmotor features of Parkinson's disease*). Here the reader will find the key areas of depression, anxiety, cognitive impairment, and dementia, amongst others. The chapter describes the clinical features of these complications and considers the drug treatments which have been tested in clinical trials and which can now be applied in clinical care.

Although much of the severity scoring for Parkinson's disease is applied in the clinical trial setting, an understanding of the assessment scales is important in the interpretation of the clinical research literature. In addition, selective application of scores and scales can be helpful in obtaining a comprehensive clinical picture. For example the identification of non-motor features such as depression, and other aspects of PD, can be made more objective with a scoring system. Where a short version of such a scoring scheme is available, we guide the reader to this alternative, to help save time in the busy clinic. We also cover the schemes that patients can administer primarily themselves, which mainly relate to functional ability and quality of life. There are therefore many reasons for including Chapter 6, *Motor and nonmotor assessment scales,* which takes a step-by-step approach and comments on the limitations and benefits of each instrument.

Chapter 6 concludes with one of the assessment tools used when considering a patient for surgery – which nowadays is mainly deep brain stimulation (DBS) surgery. DBS is the focus for Chapter 7, *Surgical therapy for Parkinson's disease*, and details of the evaluation criteria to select appropriate patients for surgical intervention are presented. Issues of cognitive screening, psychiatric co-morbidity, and any previous antiparkinson medication effects the patient has experienced are reviewed. The chapter moves on to the practical issues of the type of surgery, then onto DBS techniques such as the localization of the surgical target and the application of micro-electrode recording.

The work of allied team professionals is looked at in the following chapters. *The role of the nurse practitioner/physician assistant* (Chapter 8) emphasizes the coordination of care and communication with patient, family and other caregivers. *The role of the physical and occupational therapist* (Chapter 9) again looks beyond the simple physical limitations of the condition. The wider aspects of perceptual ability, the impact of cognitive impairments, the effect of antiparkinson medication on the patient's physical condition are all addressed, as well as different approaches to the management of a range of movements, posture, balance, and gait. The individual functions on which all this has impact are then considered from the occupational therapy point of view. In Chapter 10, *The role of the speech–language pathologist/therapist*, the Parkinson patient's specific problems with communication and swallowing are addressed. This is set against a wider background of communication and swallowing disorders and the impact of cognitive slowing and impairment, together with referral and evaluation considerations and potential treatment techniques.

In Chapter 11, *Malnutrition and related disorders*, the dietician's role is defined, with discussion of both the risk factors and identification of malnutrition, and also the management of bowel status, vitamin status, interaction with other disease features like depression, loss of sense of smell, and concerns relating to the nutritional effects of antiparkinson medication. Finally, *Complementary medicine and Parkinson's disease*, Chapter 12, examines the usefulness of complementary approaches in the management of Parkinson's, with a point-by-point review of popular therapies such as acupuncture and dietary supplementation.

A list of resources for the patient and family, as well as caregivers, is provided at the end of the book, and also a list of further reading, a glossary explaining many of the specialized terms used in the text, a list of abbreviations, and an index.

DONALD GROSSET, KATHERINE GROSSET,
HUBERT FERNANDEZ, MICHAEL OKUN

CHAPTER 1

Parkinson's disease facts and figures

History

- Parkinson's disease (PD) was first formally described by James Parkinson in an 1817 report (earlier records include a Shakespeare character with the condition).
- He described tremor, gait disorder, and brady-kinesia which he confused with paralysis, contributing to the misnomer 'paralysis agitans'.
- He was a general practitioner in Shoreditch, England.
- His observations were based on six cases – two of whom he met in the street and one of whom he had only seen from a distance.

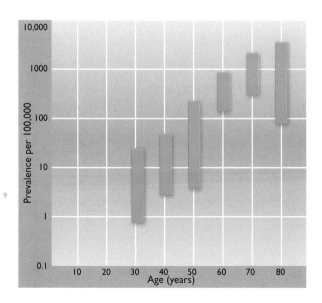

1 Prevalence of idiopathic PD by age. Prevalence increases with age. Ranges are shown from major studies which used varying methodology (specialist clinics, health records, door-to-door surveys). Note that the y axis is logarithmic: the rise per decade is exponential.

Epidemiology

- Estimating exactly how many people have PD is difficult due to inaccuracy in diagnosis.
- Between 750,000 and 1 million people in the USA and 120,000–130,000 in the UK have PD.
- There are between 4 and 20 new cases per 100,000 population per year (this incidence figure, the number of new cases in a year, is not affected by survival, but is influenced by diagnostic accuracy).
- The incidence and prevalence of PD increase with age (**1**).
- In a large population-based study in Rochester, Minnesota, the overall age-adjusted incidence of PD was relatively stable from 1979–1990. However, there was an increase for those aged 70–99 years, mainly due to drug-induced parkinsonism.
- The prevalence of PD (the total number of cases at one time point) is estimated at between 100 and 180 per 100,000. Prevalence rates across Europe vary from 66 per 100,000 in Sardinia to 12,500 per 100,000 in institutionalized patients in Germany. In the USA, crude prevalence rates vary from 100 per 100,000 in New York (community-based study) to 347 per 100,000 in Mississippi (from a door-to-door survey).
- About 2% of people over 65 years have PD.
- Prevalence statistics are affected by survival, so that in diseases such as PD, the prevalence rate is much higher than the incidence rate.
- Hospital-based studies show increasing incidence and prevalence rates with increasing age, but the rates seem to decline in older patients. Community-based studies do not show declining rates of PD with age, indicating that the hospital studies failed to identify all cases.

- The average age of onset of symptoms is approximately 60 years.
- PD is more common in Caucasians, less common in West Africa, and intermediate in China. African-Americans and the Chinese in Taiwan have higher rates of PD than their counterparts in West Africa or China, suggesting that environmental factors may play a role.
- Men have a 1.5 times greater risk of developing PD than women.
- PD is called young-onset if it occurs between the ages of 20 and 40 years, and juvenile-onset when symptoms start below 21 years of age (**2**).

Survival

- There is uncertainty about the effect of PD on survival.
- The estimated standardized mortality rate (the ratio of number of deaths in PD patients to controls) varies between 1.5 and 2.4. Follow-up of 15–18 years of 149 patients in the Sydney multi-centre study reported a standardized mortality rate of 1.86. Hoehn and Yahr (who reported in the 1960s) found a standardized mortality rate of 2.9 (95% confidence interval (CI) 2.4–3.6), but this predated levodopa therapy and there were methodological issues. The excess in mortality increased with disease duration in a recent study of survival of men with PD.

- The mean age at death was 82 years in 170 PD patients versus 83 years in 510 matched controls with 9 years' follow-up in one study.
- Only half of death certificates in PD patients include PD as an underlying condition or contributory cause. PD is not usually a direct cause of death. The primary cause of death is most commonly a secondary complication such as bronchopneumonia.
- Earlier death is associated with dementia and later disease onset.
- Although younger patients with PD have a longer absolute survival from diagnosis to death, the disease has a greater influence on survival in younger patients because of their greater life expectancy.
- Tremor-dominant patients have better survival than those without tremor.
- Tremor-dominant patients also have better survival compared to patients with postural instability and gait disturbance.
- There are pathological data suggesting degeneration of different areas in tremor-dominant versus akinetic–rigid types.
- These observations may be partly explained by diagnostic error: some tremor patients may not have true parkinsonism and will have better survival, while some akinetic–rigid patients may have a Parkinson-plus syndrome which progresses more rapidly.

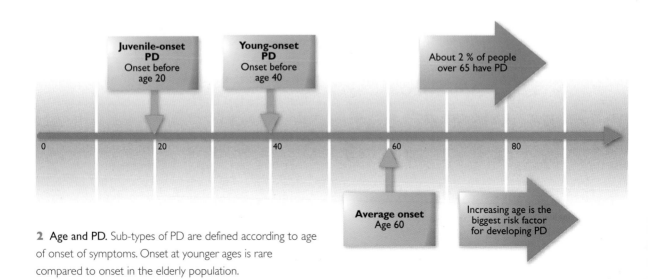

2 Age and PD. Sub-types of PD are defined according to age of onset of symptoms. Onset at younger ages is rare compared to onset in the elderly population.

Causes

- The cause of PD remains unknown.
- Genetic and environmental causes, and an interaction between environmental risk factors and genetic susceptibility are all possible.
- PD may not be a single disease entity. The clinical presentation of PD may be caused by several different conditions.
- There is depigmentation through loss of neuromelanin in the substantia nigra (**3**).
- The damage in the substantia nigra affects the nerves which project to the striatum, hence nigrostriatal pathway (**4**).
- The deterioration in nerve cells in PD occurs through a process referred to as apoptosis.
- Apoptosis means programmed cell death, which is a scheduled process of cell shrinkage and involves disposal of cell contents and remnants. Some understanding of the triggers of apoptosis has come from identifying genetic causes of PD (see below).

Risk factors

- *Increasing age* is the largest risk factor for developing PD.
- *A family history of PD* is the second most important risk factor for developing PD.
- *Higher education.* In a recent study from Rochester, Minnesota, USA, people with 9 or more years of higher education had an odds ratio of 2.0 (95% CI 1.1–3.6) of developing PD compared to those with less education.
- *Occupation.* In the Rochester study, physicians had a higher risk of developing PD, while those who worked in construction, production with metal, and engineers had reduced rates of PD (this may be a referral bias). However in a study from Alabama, USA, the prevalence of parkinsonism was higher among welders versus age-standardized data for the general population (prevalence ratio 10.2; 95% CI 4.4–23.4).
- *Head trauma.* Controversy exists as to whether a history of head trauma is a risk factor. Although there is some retrospective evidence of head trauma increasing the risk of developing PD, other studies do not confirm this association and the results may be influenced by recall bias.

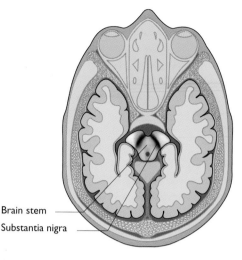

Brain stem
Substantia nigra

3 Substantia nigra. Brain section at the level of the brainstem. The face is anterior, and the lobes of the brain are shown to each side of the brainstem. The substantia nigra lies within the brainstem and is the origin of the nerves projecting to the striatum. Normal pigmentation is shown. In Parkinson's disease these areas are depigmented.

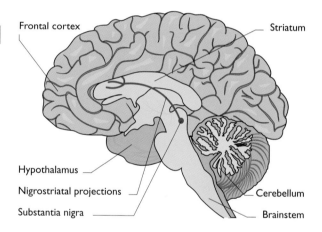

Frontal cortex — Striatum

Hypothalamus
Nigrostriatal projections — Cerebellum
Substantia nigra — Brainstem

4 Nigrostriatal pathway. Brain section approximately at the midline (lateral view). The nigrostriatal pathway connects the substantia nigra to the striatum. These nerves are sometimes described as nigrostriatal projections. Dopamine is the main neurotransmitter in this pathway.

There are no prospective studies of head trauma patients having an increased risk of developing PD. The one study which followed cases of head injury did not find any increased risk of PD. However, trauma may worsen existing symptoms in patients with known PD.

Genetic factors

◆ The majority of PD cases are sporadic, but a few are inherited (**5**).

◆ If an individual has a family history of PD, the risk of developing PD is doubled compared to the rate in the background population.

◆ Between 15 and 20% of patients have a positive family history of PD.

◆ However, the largest twin study conducted in PD concluded that genetic factors do not play a major role in causing typical PD. In this study of over 19,000 twins, there was no difference in the concordance rate for monozygotic and dizygotic twins for typical late-onset idiopathic PD, but genetic factors were important for those presenting before 50 years of age.

◆ In 16 twin pairs with diagnosis of PD at or before the age of 50 years in at least 1 twin, monozygotic concordance was 1.0 (four pairs), and dizygotic was 0.167 (relative risk 6.0; 95% CI 1.7–21.3) (**5**).

◆ Functional imaging reveals reduced basal ganglia 18-fluorodopa uptake in monozygotic twins (75% concordance) compared to dizygotic twins (22% concordance), supporting a role of genetic factors in developing PD (**5**).

◆ Gene mutations implicated in the development of PD include gene loci PARK 1 to 11. Some are autosomal dominant (AD) and others are autosomal recessive (AR) (**6**):

◇ PARK 1 (AD), located on chromosome 4q 21-q23, encodes for the protein alpha-synuclein, and is associated with Lewy bodies (the pathological hallmark of PD and Lewy body dementia). PARK 1 was first described in an Italian-American family originating from Contursi and subsequently found in several families from Greece and elsewhere. Clinically, symptom onset is at an earlier age and tremor is less likely than in classical PD.

5 Twin studies and genetic contribution to PD.
The majority of cases of PD are sporadic, and even patients with a positive family history do not have a specific genetic type of PD. Genetic types of PD help our understanding of how the disorder might develop. Twin studies give a unique insight into genetic mechanisms. Both clinical diagnosis and abnormalities in brain scanning have been studied. High concordance for monozygotic twins lends support to a genetic cause for the disorder.

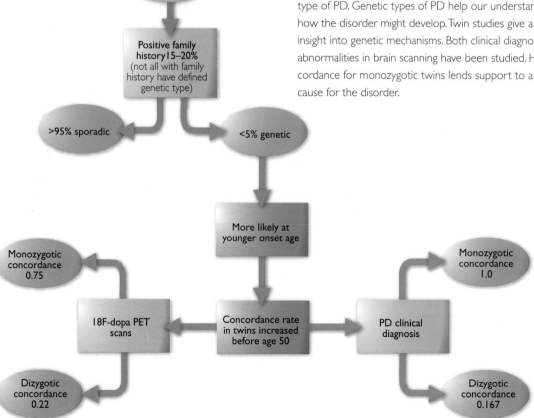

Gene mutations in Parkinson's disease

AUTOSOMAL DOMINANT

PARK 1	Codes for α-Synuclein Lewy bodies present Early onset Less likely to have tremor
PARK 3	Lewy bodies present Later onset
PARK 4	α-Synuclein expression doubled Lewy body pathology extensive Autonomic dysfunction Dementia Weight loss
PARK 8	Average onset 51 years Very similar to PD
PARK 11	Very similar to PD

AUTOSOMAL RECESSIVE

PARK 2	Codes for Parkin Lewy bodies mainly absent Early or juvenile onset More dystonia + dyskinesia
PARK 6	Codes for the PINK 1 protein Early onset Slow progression
PARK 7	Early onset Slow progression Psychiatric disturbance Dystonia (e.g. blepharospasm)
PARK 9	Unlike PD Pallido-pyramidal degeneration Supranuclear gaze paresis Dementia

UNCERTAIN INHERITANCE

PARK 5	Reported in 2 German siblings
PARK 10	Reported in 51 Icelandic families Late-onset PD

6 **Gene mutations in Parkinson's disease.** Several gene mutations have been identified, and are associated with different phenotypes of the disease. Collectively the known gene mutations account for a very small proportion of PD cases, but the variation in clinical features and progression rates illustrates a spectrum of disease that is also seen in the wider PD population.

◇ PARK 2 (AR), located on chromosome 6q25.2-q27, encodes for the parkin protein, which has a role in protein digestion (**7**). Lewy bodies are absent (only a few brains from patients with parkin mutations have been examined; Lewy bodies were absent in all but two cases). This was first described in a Japanese family and patients can have an early or juvenile onset, a symmetrical presentation, more levodopa-induced dyskinesia, and slower disease progression compared to classical PD. Excess psychiatric symptoms, early dystonia and hyperreflexia, which were previously considered to be clinical indicators of parkin-associated PD, may correlate better with younger age of onset rather than the parkin mutation. However in a recent report from China the phenotype of slow progression, diurnal variation with sleep

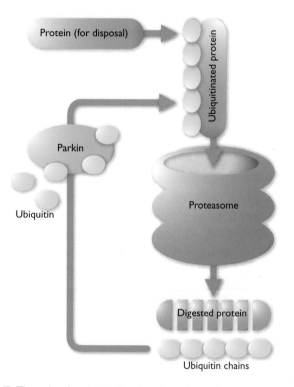

7 **The role of parkin in the digestion of protein.**
Parkin has a role in faciliitating the attachment of ubiquitin to protein which is scheduled for disposal. Protein is ubiquitinated before it passes through the proteasome and becomes digested. The ubiquitin chains are then disconnected from the digested protein and recycled.

benefit and hyperreflexia was relatively prominent. Mutations in parkin account for around 50% of AR young-onset familial PD and should be considered in cases with a family history consistent with recessive inheritance and disease onset before the age of 45. In 'parkin disease' PET (positive emission tomography) confirms presynaptic dopamine deficiency but, unlike classical PD, the severity of the PET abnormality does not correlate with the clinical features (see Chapter 3).

◇ PARK 3 (AD) is located on chromosome 2p13 and is associated with later onset (average age 59 years), cognitive impairment, and levodopa responsiveness. Lewy bodies are present. It has been identified in kindreds from northern Europe.

◇ PARK 4 (AD) has now been mapped to PARK 1 (chromosome 4q21). Individuals have doubling of alpha-synuclein expression (there is a triplication of the alpha-synuclein gene giving four copies of the usual gene rather than two) and more extensive Lewy body pathology. Clinically, autonomic dysfunction, dementia, and weight loss occur in conjunction with parkinsonism.

◇ PARK 5 (possibly AD). There is a mutation in the gene encoding ubiquitin carboxy-terminal hydrolase L1 (UCH-L1) – this has only been reported in two German siblings who have a missense mutation in this gene and may be an extremely rare form of familial PD with incomplete penetrance. However since the original report of these two cases in 1998, there have been no other kindreds with this mutation (193M in the UCH-L1 gene). A more recent report suggests that UCH-L1 is not a PD susceptibility gene.

◇ PARK 6 (AR), located on chromosome 1p35-p36, encodes for the PINK 1 protein and is associated with early age of onset and slower disease progression. It was first identified in an Italian family from Sicily from which four family members developed PD between the ages of 32 and 48 years. Functional imaging using PET shows a more uniform pattern of reduced uptake in the caudate and putamen and a greater degree of dopamine loss than would be expected from the clinical severity.

The PINK 1 protein protects against stress-induced mitochondrial dysfunction and apotosis.

◇ PARK 7 (AR) is located on chromosome 1p36 and is associated with early onset, slow disease progression, psychiatric disturbance, and dystonic features (e.g. blepharospasm). There is a mutation in the DJ-1 gene and cells lacking in DJ-1 appear to be more susceptible to oxidative stress.

◇ PARK 8 (AD) is located on chromosome 12p11.2-q13.1. The average age of onset is 51 years and clinical signs are very similar to those of typical PD, with unilateral onset and levodopa responsiveness. Foot dystonia may be present prior to and during drug therapy. Overall, patients do not report drug-induced dyskinesia. Functional imaging with 18F-dopa PET shows the same pattern of nigro-striatal dysfunction that is seen in PD (i.e. preferential degeneration of the posterior dorsal putamen with relative sparing of the anterior dorsal putamen and head of caudate). Pathology is variable; one case from the Lincolnshire kindred in the UK had loss of the pigmented neurones and gliosis of the substantia nigra and typical Lewy bodies. However, nigral degeneration without Lewy bodies was reported in the original description from Japan. A novel gene LRRK2 (leucine-rich, repeat kinase 2), which encodes for the protein dardarin, has been identified as the gene responsible. The frequency of LRRK2 mutation is around 5% in cases of familial PD (based on a series of 118 familial PD patients: patients with one or more affected first-degree relatives) and 1–2% in sporadic PD.

◇ PARK 9 (AR). The phenotype is unlike PD. Features are of pallido-pyramidal degeneration, supranuclear gaze paresis, and dementia.

◇ PARK 10 (unknown inheritance pattern). 51 Icelandic families were genotyped and a susceptibility locus for late-onset PD was identified.

◇ PARK 11 (AD). This locus was identified from genome-wide linkage analysis in a large multicentre study in the USA. No definite phenotype or inheritance is reported.

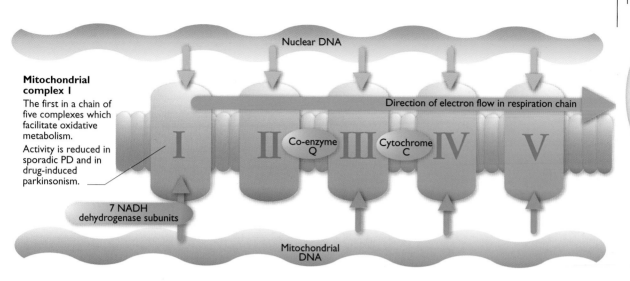

Mitochondrial complex I
The first in a chain of five complexes which facilitate oxidative metabolism.
Activity is reduced in sporadic PD and in drug-induced parkinsonism.

Nuclear DNA

Direction of electron flow in respiration chain

I   II   Co-enzyme Q   III   Cytochrome C   IV   V

7 NADH dehydrogenase subunits

Mitochondrial DNA

8 Mitochondrial complexes. There are five complexes within the mitochondrial electron transport chain, of which a deficiency has been found in the first, mitochondrial complex I, in sporadic PD, as well as in experimental models of drug-induced (MPTP and rotenone) parkinsonism.

◆ Mitochondrial inheritance:
   ◇ A deficiency of mitochondrial complex I has been found which may be caused by a mitochondrial gene defect (**8**).
   ◇ Transmission through the maternal line was considered likely (as mitochondrial genes are maternally inherited).
   ◇ In two separate studies, however, probands were more likely to report an affected father than an affected mother (which is clearly contrary to maternal inheritance).
   ◇ Several of the gene defects identified for familial PD involve mitochondria either directly or indirectly (e.g. alpha-synuclein, parkin, DJ-1, PINK1, LRRK2).

Environmental factors

Parkinsonism can occur as a result of a range of environmental factors (**9**):
◆ Toxins:
   ◇ Heavy metals. Manganese poisoning produces parkinsonism, but the clinical and pathological features are different from idiopathic PD. In manganese intoxication early psychiatric problems (mental irritability, compulsive actions and hallucinations) occur, dystonia is more frequent, and tremor tends to be postural.

Possible environmental triggers for Parkinson's Disease

TOXINS

MANGANESE
Workers (miners, welders) exposed to manganese can develop manganese-induced parkinsonism.

PESTICIDES AND SOLVENTS
Carbon disulphide, used in pesticides and solvents, can cause parkinsonism. Other chemicals can be similarly toxic. Increased risk in rural areas (use of well water).

CARBON MONOXIDE
Exposure can cause delayed parkinsonism. Bradykinesia, rigidity and occasional resting tremor. Dystonia and emotional changes may be present.

MPTP
A contaminant of 'street' heroin. Users developed severe parkinsonism, which was non-progressive.

VIRUSES

Post-encephalitic parkinsonism. Infective, probably viral etiology. Major outbreak in 1920s.

TRAUMA

Post-traumatic parkinsonism (punch-drunk syndrome). Head injury features in cross-sectional studies of PD. Not corroborated by prospective study (may represent recall bias).

9 Environmental causes of PD. Several potential environmental toxins have been implicated in PD. However, for the majority of patients, there is no identifiable external trigger for the development of their condition.

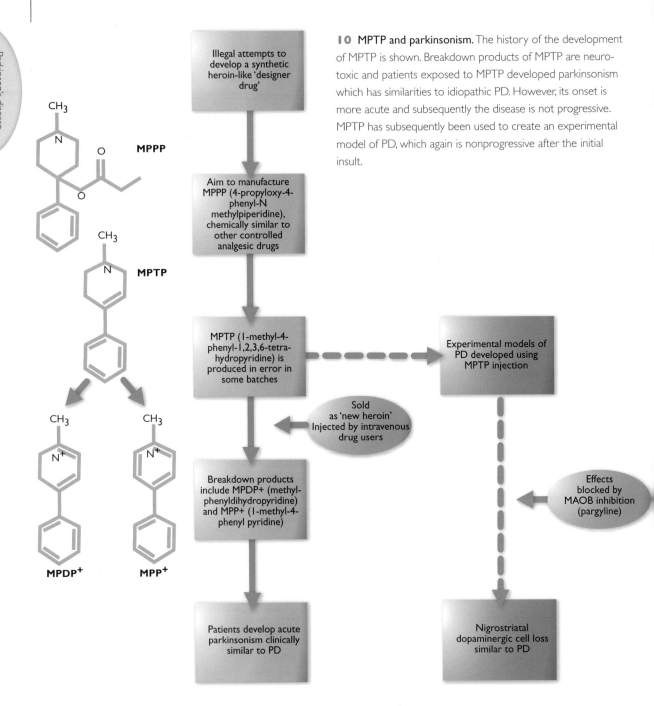

10 MPTP and parkinsonism. The history of the development of MPTP is shown. Breakdown products of MPTP are neurotoxic and patients exposed to MPTP developed parkinsonism which has similarities to idiopathic PD. However, its onset is more acute and subsequently the disease is not progressive. MPTP has subsequently been used to create an experimental model of PD, which again is nonprogressive after the initial insult.

◇ People living in Guam who consumed water containing aluminium and had low dietary intake of magnesium and calcium developed a parkinsonism–dementia complex. A separate theory suggested that the syndrome was caused by a plant neurotoxin from cycad flour.

◇ MPTP (1-methyl-4-phenyl-1,2,3,6-tetrahydropyridine). A chemistry graduate in San Francisco manufactured a pethidine analogue for street sale which was contaminated with MPTP (**10**). Intravenous drug users injecting this product developed severe parkinsonism and active neuronal loss was found at autopsy (although many survived).

◇ Compounds structurally similar to MPTP are found in pesticides; small case–control studies show a small increased risk of parkinsonism in rural areas and farms, and in those who drink well water, but population-based controlled studies fail to show any association.

◇ Iron may enhance free radical formation causing lipid peroxidation and cell death.

◇ Carbon monoxide. Parkinsonism is a delayed effect of carbon monoxide toxicity and has features of bradykinesia, rigidity, and occasional resting tremor. Dystonia and emotional changes may also be present. Another variant is of akinetic mutism.

◆ Infections. In the early 1900s post-encephalitic parkinsonism raised the possibility of an infective (probably viral) aetiology. The acute phase of the disease usually lasts several weeks and the clinical picture is of pronounced somnolence and ophthalmoplegia. The parkinsonian syndrome presents months or years later (median 5 years). However, the clinical and pathological features of post-encephalitic parkinsonism are different from those of idiopathic PD. In post-encephalitic parkinsonism clinical progression is slow and pathologically there are Alzheimer-type neurofibrillary tangles, whereas PD is a progressive disorder and histologically there are Lewy bodies.

◆ Emotional stress. An increased risk of PD has been reported in people who have endured extreme psychological and physical stress. It is postulated that emotional stress increases dopamine turnover causing oxidative nerve cell death. This is unproven.

◆ Personality. Premorbid personality traits of shyness, being more introverted, and depression have been associated with an increased risk of PD. In retrospective studies PD patients were more cautious, less flexible, and quieter compared to control subjects. This needs to be examined in larger studies.

Protective factors

◆ Cigarette smoking is protective against the development of PD (**11**).

◆ A review of all observational studies evaluating the association between PD risk and a smoking habit found an obvious protective effect of smoking. The risk estimate was 0.37 (95% CI 0.33–0.41, i.e. the risk of developing PD as a cigarette smoker is reduced to about one-third that of non-smokers).

◆ Former smokers versus those who have never smoked have a risk estimate of 0.84 (95% CI 0.76–0.92).

◆ This protective effect remains even after correction for smoking-related mortality.

◆ Proposed explanations include:

◇ Protective effects of nicotine.

◇ Personality factors – the 'parkinsonian personality' who avoids certain novelty-seeking behaviours such as cigarette smoking; or there may be a change in personality in the preclinical phase of PD associated with a reduced likelihood of continuing or starting smoking. An alternative theory suggests there may be smoking cessation due to olfactory loss known to coexist with PD.

◆ Vitamins C and E are possibly associated with PD but prospective evidence is lacking. In meta-analysis, dietary vitamin E was possibly marginally protective and vitamin C and betacarotene had no effect.

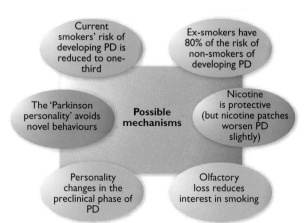

11 Cigarette smoking and the risk of Parkinson's disease. Cigarette smoking is protective to the risk of PD and possible mechanisms are illustrated.

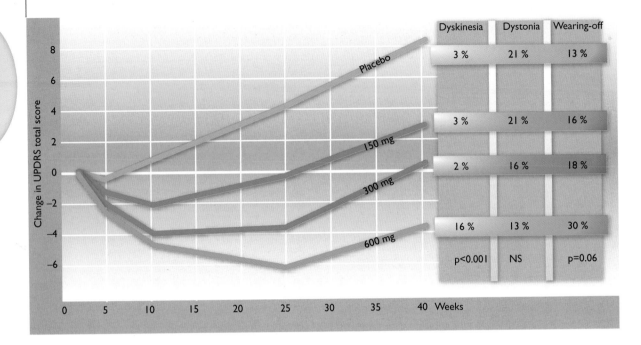

	Dyskinesia	Dystonia	Wearing-off
Placebo	3 %	21 %	13 %
150 mg	3 %	21 %	16 %
300 mg	2 %	16 %	18 %
600 mg	16 %	13 %	30 %
	p<0.001	NS	p=0.06

Disease progression

◆ Clinical signs and symptoms develop once there is at least 50% depletion of striatal dopamine (estimated from imaging studies). However there may be as much as 60–80% loss of pigmented neurones in the substantia nigra (compensatory mechanisms may affect the scan appearance and thereby account for the discrepancy, see Chapter 3).

◆ The preclinical phase of the disease may be 1 to several years but this is unknown.

◆ The rates of disease progression vary between individuals.

◆ Some tremor-dominant patients progress very slowly, which is sometimes termed 'benign tremulous Parkinson's'.

◆ 10–20% of patients have no tremor and remain akinetic–rigid or primarily have a gait disorder.

◆ When patients commence treatment, there is usually an improvement in the motor function score. The response to levodopa is dose-related (e.g. in the ELLDOPA study patients randomized to the highest levodopa dose had the greatest improvement in motor scores, **12**). In a 5-year follow-up study comparing immediate versus sustained-release co-carbidopa, the New York University Parkinson Disease Scale of disability improved initially, then slowly declined until it reached baseline levels at 5 years for both treatment groups. Clinical improvements,

12 The ELLDOPA study. This compared different doses of levodopa with placebo. The greatest improvement in motor score occurred at the highest doses, but this was associated with greater risk of motor complications, in particular dyskinesia.

measured by the unified PD rating scale (UPDRS) motor score (see Chapter 6), tend to be better with levodopa than with dopamine agonists, e.g. in the REAL-PET study after 2 years the UPDRS motor score had deteriorated by 0.7 (standard error 0.97) in the ropinirole group compared to an improvement of 5.64 (standard error 1.05) in the levodopa group.

◆ In untreated patients (e.g. in the DATATOP trial, which compared placebo against selegiline (deprenyl) and/or vitamin E) the total UPDRS score deteriorated by 13 points per year.

◆ Motor complications (wearing off, involuntary movements, and the 'on'/'off' effect) are traditionally stated to occur in 50% of patients after 5 years on levodopa treatment, although lower rates than this are described in several studies. In general, DA (dopamine agonist) monotherapy is associated with lower motor complication rates.

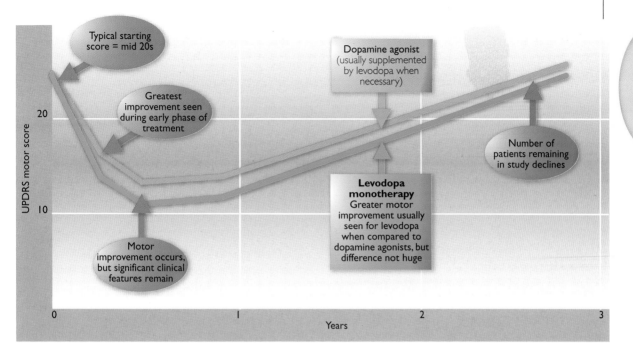

13 Comparison of dopamine agonists and levodopa therapy. In general a greater motor improvement is seen for levodopa. Improvement in motor score is good particularly initially but there is residual motor deficit despite optimization of oral treatment. In later stages beyond the original end-point of the study, the numbers remaining under observation decline so that conclusions are less definite about long-term comparison of these drug classes.

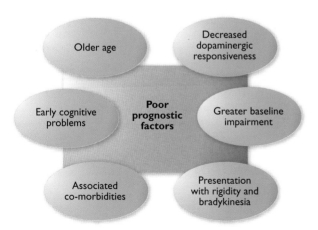

14 Prognosis. The factors relating to poor prognosis in PD are shown.

◆ For patients on levodopa 40% remain free of dyskinesia after 5 years, versus 70% who are free of dyskinesia if on DA treatment. However, levodopa is a more efficacious treatment in terms of improvement in motor score (**13**).

◆ Young-onset patients (<40 years) develop motor complications earlier, occurring in almost 100% at 6 years.

◆ Patients who are older at symptom onset generally have a more rapid deterioration in motor features (based on a recent population-based cohort study of 232 patients from Norway).

◆ Functional imaging studies suggest an annual loss of 8% (range 6–11%) of presynaptic dopamine transporters versus 0.3–1% per year through ageing (see Chapter 3).

◆ Pathological studies show similar results with eight to ten times accelerated nigral degeneration compared with healthy age-matched controls.

◆ Older age, early cognitive problems, associated co-morbidities, presentation with rigidity and bradykinesia (i.e. lack of tremor at onset), decreased dopamine responsiveness, and greater baseline impairment are associated with poorer prognosis (**14**).

◆ Progression of disease may not be linear. Several studies suggest that the rate of decline is more rapid initially, then slows in the more advanced disease stages (however, the effects of treatment need to be considered, as this will influence interpretation of severity and progression rates).

Pathophysiology

◆ Pathways for initiating motor movement run from the premotor and motor cortex, via the striatum and globus pallidus (GP) to the thalamus, which feeds back to the cortex. There is a highly organized network of multiple cortical loops, 'internal' circuits, and microcircuits.

◆ These 'loops' within brain circuitry modulate motor output through several neuronal connections (**15**).

◆ The striatum has two inhibitory projections to the GP, one of which is a direct pathway and the other is indirect (**15**).

◇ The direct pathway connects the striatum directly to the medial (or internal) GP (GPi).

◇ The indirect pathway connects initially to the lateral (or external) GP (GPe), then to the subthalamic nucleus (STN), and finally back to the GPi.

◇ Activation of the direct pathway uses the D1 dopamine receptor system, and is inhibitory. D5 is very similar to D1 and the two are referred to as D1-like (**16**).

◇ Activation of the indirect pathway uses the D2 subtype of dopamine neurones, and the overall effect is excitatory. D3 and D4 are similar to D2, though there are some differences in affinity for dopamine (D3) and clozapine, an antipsychotic, which is highly selective at D4 (**16**).

◇ Increased activity of the GPi and STN inhibits movement, while inhibition of these areas facilitates movement.

◇ In health, a balance between direct and indirect pathways promotes fine, organized motor activity.

15 Basal ganglia circuitry. Connections between motor cortex and components of the basal ganglia are shown. Dotted lines represent inhibitory flow and solid lines represent excitatory flow. The primary defect in PD is loss of nigrostriatal dopamine (i.e. the neural pathway between the substantia nigra and the striatum [1]). D1 and D2 refer to dopamine receptor subtypes (further dopamine receptor subtypes are explained in 16).

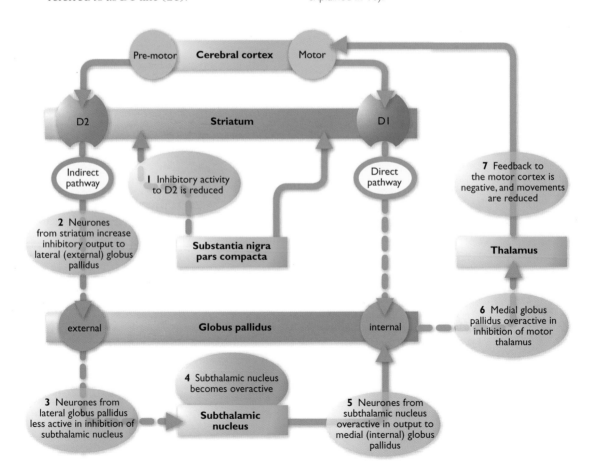

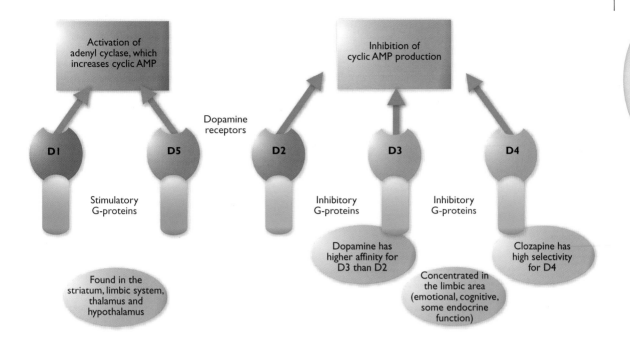

In PD there is degeneration of the dopaminergic neurones in the pars compacta of the substantia nigra.

The loss of dopaminergic neurones leads to reduced inhibition of the indirect neurones and less inhibition from the decreased activity of the GPe; there is thus increased activity in the STN and increased stimulation of the GPi via the indirect pathway, and diminished inhibition (therefore hyperactivity) of the GPi via the direct pathway as shown in **15**. This, in turn, over-inhibits the motor projections to the thalamus and brainstem.

The STN and the GPi have neuronal hyperactivity and are therefore sites for surgical intervention in PD (see Chapter 7). There is overinhibition of the motor thalamus (the surgical site used to diminish tremor) and brainstem nuclei. Lesioning these areas damages the overactive area, and helps restore normal (positive) motor outputs. A lesion in the STN reduces the excess stimulation of the GPi, and decreases inhibition of the thalamocorti-cal neurones. A lesion of the GPi reduces excessive inhibition of the thalamocortical neurones.

◇ The placement of stimulators – which deliver an electrical current causing functional blockade – has a similar effect (see Chapter 7).

16 Dopamine receptor subtypes. There are two main groupings, the D1 and D1-like dopamine receptor subtypes and the D2 and D2-like dopamine receptor subtypes. The D1 agents (stimulatory G-proteins) activate adenyl cyclase – the enzyme which synthesizes the AMP messenger system – while D2 agents (inhibitory G-proteins) reduce its activity. Further characteristics of dopamine receptor subtypes D3 and D4 are as shown.

Chorea (writhing, rotatory movements with jumps) and ballism (flinging or throwing movements, typically of one arm) are positive involuntary movements which were thought to be induced by the opposite mechanism: overac-tivity of the direct pathway, and underactivity of the GPi and STN. However, several clinical and experimental findings do not fit with this explana-tion, e.g. lesioning or functional blockade of the STN does not lead to chorea or ballism.

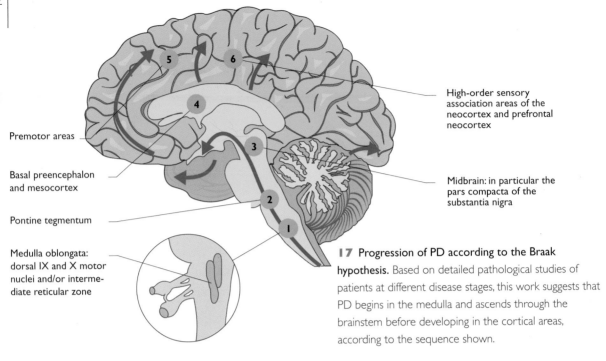

High-order sensory association areas of the neocortex and prefrontal neocortex

Premotor areas

Basal preencephalon and mesocortex

Pontine tegmentum

Medulla oblongata: dorsal IX and X motor nuclei and/or intermediate reticular zone

Midbrain: in particular the pars compacta of the substantia nigra

17 **Progression of PD according to the Braak hypothesis.** Based on detailed pathological studies of patients at different disease stages, this work suggests that PD begins in the medulla and ascends through the brainstem before developing in the cortical areas, according to the sequence shown.

Neuropathology

◆ In PD there is neuronal death in the pars compacta of the substantia nigra (see **3**).
  ◇ These neurones are pigmented as they contain neuromelanin, which is subsequently removed from the dead cells by microglia.
  ◇ This results in depigmentation which can be seen histologically.
◆ Histologically specific inclusion bodies develop: spindle- or thread-like (Lewy neurites) or in a globular form (Lewy bodies – intracytoplasmic eosinophilic areas with a densely staining core, surrounding halo, and a larger outer body). These are traditionally considered the prerequisite for the postmortem diagnosis of PD (but are sometimes absent in genetic forms of PD – see above).
  ◇ Lewy neurites and Lewy bodies contain the protein alpha-synuclein.
◆ In addition to nigral damage (to the substantia nigra and its neuronal projections), there is extra-nigral damage including pathological changes in the dorsal motor nucleus of the glossopharyngeal and vagal nerves, adjoining intermediate reticular zone, some subnuclei of the reticular formation and raphe system, the coeruleus–subcoeruleus complex, the magnocellular nuclei of the forebrain, many subnuclei of the thalamus and amygdala, and, in severe cases, lesions reaching the neocortex.

◆ Braak suggests that the neuronal damage follows a predetermined sequence in which the anatomical distribution of lesions is more important than the degree of involvement. The dorsal IX and X motor nuclei in the brainstem and the anterior olfactory nucleus are the first structures to be involved (**17**). The brainstem pathology takes an upward course leading to cortical then neocortical involvement.
◆ Braak proposed 6 stages of brain pathology related to sporadic PD:
  ◇ Stage 1 – involvement confined to the medulla oblongata (inclusion bodies confined to the dorsal IX and X and/or intermediate reticular zone).
  ◇ Stage 2 – medulla oblongata and pontine tegmentum.
  ◇ Stage 3 – stage 2 plus midbrain, in particular the pars compacta of the substantia nigra.
  ◇ Stage 4 – stage 3 plus basal proencephalon and mesocortex.
  ◇ Stage 5 – stage 4 plus lesions in high-order sensory association areas of the neocortex and prefrontal neocortex.
  ◇ Stage 6 – stage 5 plus premotor areas.
◆ It is important to note that the substantia nigra is not the first structure to develop PD-related lesions and is only involved once stage 3 is reached (thus sectioning of the substantia nigra is not sufficient for neuropathological evaluation of doubtful, or early, cases).

◆ Lewy bodies are not present in some genetic forms of PD (they are mainly absent in PARK 2 PD, but these cases with young-onset genetic PD may be considered not to have idiopathic PD, see **6**).

◆ Lewy bodies occur in smaller numbers with ageing and with other neurodegenerative disorders, e.g. Lewy body dementia.

Causes of neurone death

◆ Mitochondrial dysfunction and oxidative stress.

  ◇ Mitochondrial dysfunction and oxidative stress may be important in neuronal death in PD.

  ◇ In oxidative stress there is an abnormal increase in the formation of free radicals.

  ◇ Free radicals contain unpaired electrons and are highly reactive, oxidizing other substances by extracting an electron. Free radicals may have deleterious effects on DNA and adversely affect cell function.

  ◇ Respiring cells are exposed to free radicals but there are scavenging systems present to protect respiring cells.

  ◇ There is evidence of reduced glutathione (GSH) in PD (see chapter 12). GSH is an antioxidant and a reduced level is indirect evidence of oxidative stress.

  ◇ There is an increase in nigral iron in PD. Iron accumulation augments the formation of free radicals.

◆ Evidence of mitochondrial dysfunction in PD:

  ◇ There is defective mitochondrial function following exposure to MPTP, which is used to create an experimental model of PD (see **10**). MPTP is a protoxin which is converted by a mitochondrial enzyme to MPP+ (1-methyl-4-phenylpyridine), which may inhibit the activity of complex I in oxidative phosphorylation (some pesticides and herbicides may contain substances which inhibit complex I activity; rotenone, the classical inhibitor of complex I, was once used as an insecticide). There is evidence of loss of complex I in the substantia nigra in PD. Complex I is an electron-transfer complex (see **8**) and mitochondrial function is adversely affected. Mitochondrial respiration decreases causing protean adverse reactions including a leakage of free radicals.

  ◇ Mitochondrial respiratory failure and oxidative stress are closely related; it is unclear which comes first but once one of these processes takes place, the other is induced, setting up a vicious cycle.

◆ Protein mishandling with an accumulation of alpha-synuclein has also been implicated in the death of dopaminergic neurones.

Clinical diagnosis of parkinsonism and tremor

Symptom development

◆ Symptoms of PD develop after the reserve capacity of dopaminergic neurones is exhausted. Recent [18F] fluorodopa PET studies suggest that this probably occurs after at least 50% of dopaminergic neurones have degenerated, lower than previous estimates of 60–80%. However enhanced synthesis of dopamine in surviving neurones (upregulation of striatal dopa decarboxylase activity) and increased dopaminergic stimulation of the striatum may underestimate the true proportion of cell loss.

◆ Symptoms may be present for some time (occasionally years) before the diagnosis is made, particularly in younger patients.

◆ Abnormalities in presynaptic dopamine turnover or dopamine transporter levels are detectable on functional imaging (see Chapter 3).

◆ Patients usually lose their sense of smell in the preclinical phase of PD (olfactory dysfunction is found in 70–100% of PD patients and is therefore as common as tremor).
  ◇ Olfactory dysfunction also occurs in dementia with Lewy bodies (DLB).
  ◇ Olfaction remains normal in progressive supranuclear palsy (PSP), corticobasal degeneration, and vascular parkinsonism.
  ◇ In multiple system atrophy (MSA), spinocerebellar syndromes, and essential tremor (ET), any olfactory disturbance is mild.
  ◇ Olfactory loss is usually not volunteered by the patient, who may only realize it once asked or with testing.
  ◇ Olfactory loss tends not to occur in one of the genetic types of PD (LRRK2) – see Chapter 1 for more details on this type of PD.

◆ A higher rate of PD is reported in patients with ET, and in families with ET, than for the general public, but quantifying the relationship is difficult.
  ◇ A recent study using functional imaging suggests two separate entities.
  ◇ ET is relatively common, so inevitably some patients with ET will later develop PD.
  ◇ Rarely, ET occurs in conjunction with familial PD.
  ◇ A subset of patients presents temporally with ET and PD.

Clinical features

◆ The three cardinal features of PD (**18**) are:
  ◇ Bradykinesia (see page 28).
  ◇ Muscular rigidity (see page 31).
  ◇ Tremor (4–6 Hz rest tremor) (see page 32).

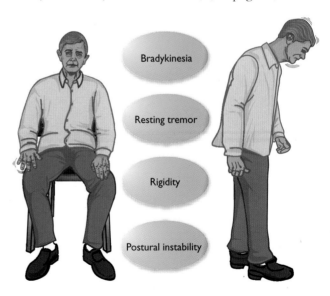

18 Cardinal features of PD. These represent Step 1 of the diagnostic criteria. Bradykinesia is a definite requirement for the diagnosis along with at least one of the other features.

◆ To reach a diagnosis of PD, there must be bradykinesia and at a least one of the two other cardinal features (this forms step 1 of the UK Parkinson's Disease Brain Bank criteria).

◆ Postural instability (not caused by primary visual, vestibular, cerebellar or proprioceptive dysfunction) is often included as a fourth or supporting feature. It is also an inclusion criterion in step 1 of the UK Parkinson's Disease Brain Bank criteria.

◆ Diagnostic criteria form a useful framework for clinical and research activities.

◆ The UK Brain Bank criteria were developed from an autopsy study of 100 cases carrying a PD diagnosis (**19**).

  ◇ Alternative diagnoses were identified in 24% of cases, including cases of PSP, MSA, and lacunar cerebrovascular disease.

19 Brain Bank Study. Flow chart of the eventual diagnosis for 100 patients in the classic UK Brain Bank Study (1992) diagnosed clinically as PD, and in whom alternative diagnoses were found.

◇ Cases with PD confirmed at autopsy often had additional brain pathology, including cerebrovascular disease within and outwith the striatum and/or Alzheimer-type changes.

◇ A subsequent updated Brain Bank Study showed improvement in accuracy to 90% (i.e. error rate 10%) (**20**). MSA was the commonest error, being present in six out of ten cases, while two had PSP, one had post-encephalitic parkinsonism, and one had vascular parkinsonism. Assessing post-mortem diagnosis against clinical criteria shows good positive predictive values (90–93%) for several criteria, but increasing the stringency of criteria lowers diagnostic sensitivity (from 90% to 67%). The practical clinical significance is that a patient may still have PD, even if they do not completely fulfil diagnostic criteria.

◇ Accuracy against baseline or early clinical diagnosis (rather than last antemortem diagnosis) is lower.

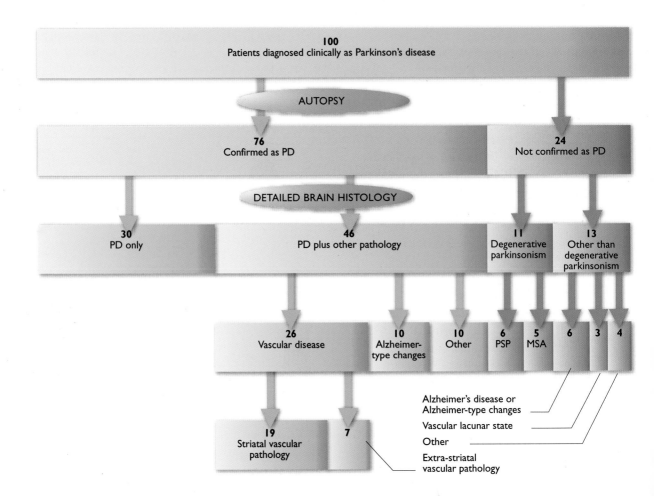

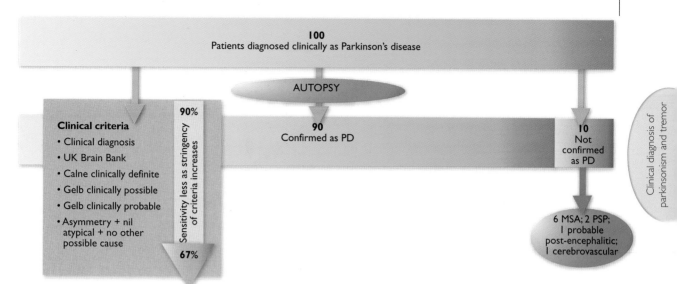

20 Brain Bank Study update. Repeat of the Brain Bank Study found improved diagnostic accuracy. Assessing the predictive value and sensitivity of different clinical assessment techniques found a fairly constant positive predictive value (90–93%) but that the sensitivity of a PD diagnosis falls as the stringency of the clinical criteria is increased.

- Step 2 of the UK Brain Bank criteria lists exclusions (**21**):
  - History of stepwise repeated strokes with stepwise progression of parkinsonian features.
  - History of repeated head injury.
  - History of definite encephalitis.
  - Oculogyric crisis.
  - Neuroleptic treatment at onset of symptoms.
  - More than one affected relative.
  - Sustained remission.
  - Strictly unilateral features after 3 years.
  - Supranuclear gaze palsy.
  - Cerebellar signs.
  - Early severe autonomic involvement.
  - Early severe dementia (disturbed memory, language, and praxis).
  - Babinski sign positive (i.e. extensor plantar response).
  - Tumour or communicating hydrocephalus on computed tomography (CT) or magnetic resonance imaging (MRI) of the brain.
  - Negative response to large doses of levodopa (if malabsorption excluded).
  - MPTP exposure.

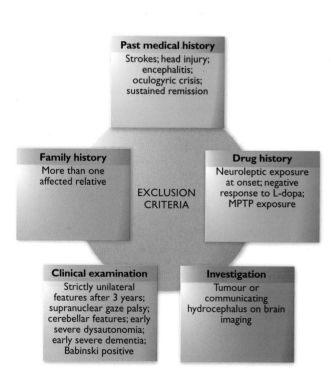

21 Brain Bank Study: Step 2. Features which reduce the likelihood of a diagnosis of idiopathic PD are shown. In practice a patient may have one of these features and still have a PD diagnosis, but they are a useful framework for considering alternative causes for parkinsonism.

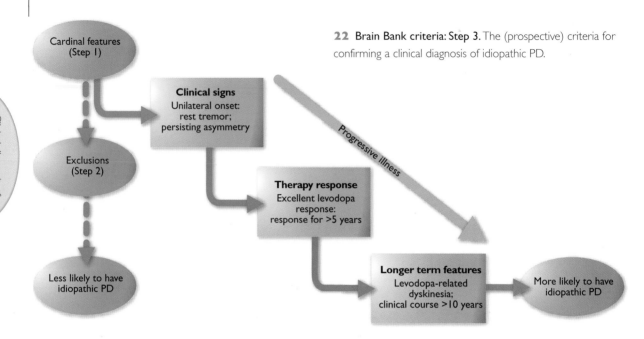

22 Brain Bank criteria: Step 3. The (prospective) criteria for confirming a clinical diagnosis of idiopathic PD.

◆ Step 3 of the UK Brain Bank criteria lists features supporting a diagnosis of PD, several of which are prospective (**22**). Three or more of the supporting criteria are required for diagnosis of definite PD.

◇ Unilateral onset.
◇ Rest tremor present.
◇ Progressive disorder.
◇ Persisting asymmetry affecting onset side most.
◇ Excellent (70–100%) response to levodopa.
◇ Severe levodopa-induced chorea.
◇ Levodopa response for at least 5 years.
◇ Clinical course of over 10 years.

◆ In clinical practice, a patient may fail Brain Bank criteria but still have PD, e.g. a patient on neuroleptic treatment who then develops idiopathic PD.

Asymmetry

◆ Idiopathic PD is generally an asymmetric condition.
◆ The side of onset (left or right) does not have an association with a patient's hemisphere dominance (i.e. handedness).
◆ Symptoms and signs remain worse on the side of onset throughout the disease course (including severity of motor fluctuations and dyskinesias).

Bradykinesia

◆ Bradykinesia is a slowness of initiating voluntary movement and sustaining repetitive movements with progressive reduction in speed and amplitude.
◆ Hypokinesia is poverty of movement.
◆ Patient symptoms and functional limitations which reflect bradykinesia/hypokinesia include:

◇ Loss of arm swing.
◇ Difficulty with walking, a tendency to drag a leg in early disease.
◇ Increasingly small handwriting (micrographia) (**23**).
◇ Difficulty with fine hand movements – buttons, zips, and cutting food.
◇ Difficulty turning in bed.
◇ Loss of facial expression, often described as a mask-like face (hypomimia) (**24**).
◇ Hypophonia (reduced voice volume and modulation) – see also Chapter 10.

23 Handwriting in PD and other tremor disorders.
(a) Micrographia, reduced letter size which worsens throughout the sentence, is a classic feature of PD.
(b) Tremulous handwriting in ET – the patient was previously diagnosed as PD and prescribed levodopa for over 1 year without benefit. Writing is shaky but does not deteriorate.

(c) Tremor in writer's cramp, a form of dystonia. This 40 year-old male had two prior self-limiting episodes of neck dystonia (spasmodic torticollis). Involuntary flexion at the wrist was associated with a high-frequency finger and thumb tremor.
(d) Cerebellar tremor. This 65-year-old male also had cerebellar dysarthria and gait ataxia. Words are ill-formed from the start of the sentence.

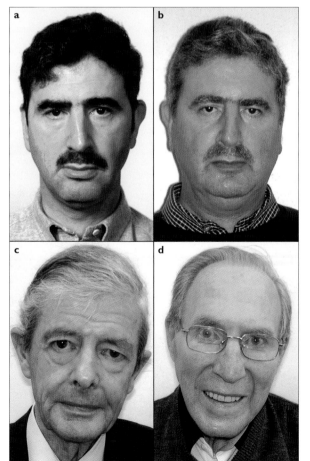

24 Loss of facial expression (hypomimia).
(a) Reduced facial expressiveness can initially be subtle and may even be evident only on one side of the face (right side in this patient) matching the unilateral limb involvement of early disease.
(b) The same patient is shown 10 years later, when features are established and bilateral.
(c) Sometimes reduced facial expressiveness could pass for a normal 'poker face'.
(d) In late disease loss of facial expression is obvious, there is a staring expression and the lips may be parted, possibly associated with salivary drooling.

- Bradykinesia/akinesia is tested clinically as follows (**25**):
  - ◇ Overall observation of slowness of spontaneous movements during the consultation.
  - ◇ Observing walking, looking for a shuffling short-steppage gait, sometimes with difficulty initiating walking (start hesitation).
  - ◇ Testing repetitive hand movements and looking for loss of amplitude, slowing or fatiguing of the action and arrests in movement: opening and closing of the hands, rapid pronation and supination at the wrist, finger taps (asking the patient to tap the index finger on the thumb repeatedly).
  - ◇ Asking the patient to tap their heel 8 cm (3 inches) from the ground repetitively.

- Bradykinesia causes significant disability affecting quality of life in PD patients and almost always responds to antiparkinsonian therapy.

25 Bradykinesia testing. Bradykinesia can be assessed from the global appearance of the patient walking and sitting in a chair (a, b), e.g. there are reduced spontaneous movements. In early disease this is more apparent in the affected body side, which is randomly the right or left side of the body (early asymmetrical PD). Testing finger, hand, and arm movements (c), as well as leg movements (d), gives additional information on the laterality of bradykinesia and the degree of slowness. Crucial to the understanding of bradykinesia is a failure to perform repetitive movements, which tend to break down. This is particularly the case when more than one movement is attempted simultaneously.

OBSERVATION
a) Walking
- Short steppage
- Dragging of one leg
- Reduced arm swing

b) Face and voice
- Loss of expression (hypomimia)
- Reduced blink rate
- Reduced voice modulation

TESTING
c) Hand and arm movements
- Opposition of index finger and thumb
- All fingers opening and closing
- Hand rotation
- Forearm rotation

d) Leg movements
- Elevation of foot at 90° to ankle

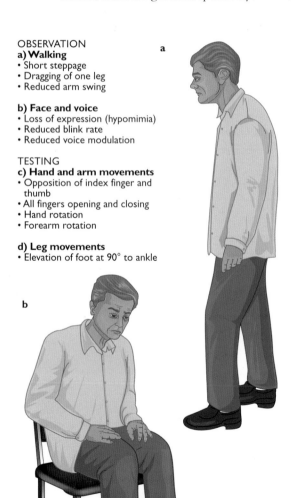
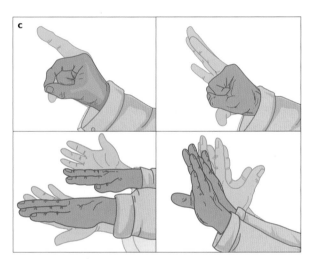
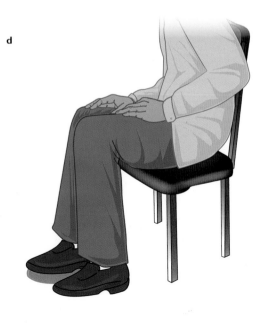

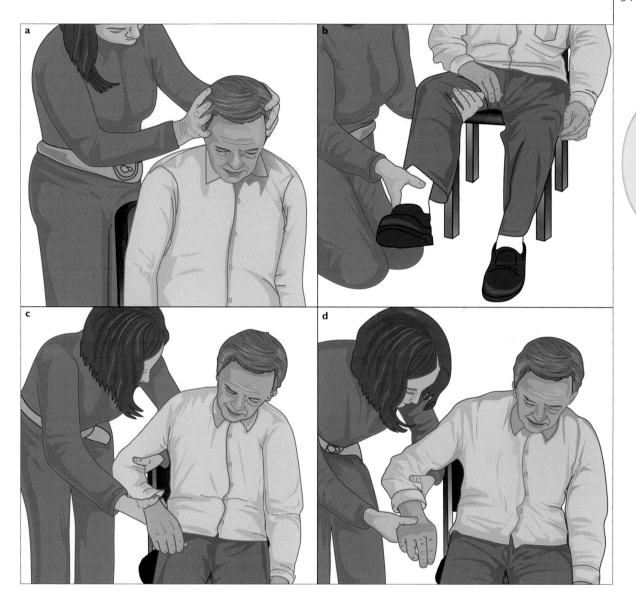

Rigidity

◆ Rigidity (**26**) is an involuntary increase in muscle tone and can affect all muscle groups. Rigidity is present throughout the range of movement and can be described as 'lead-pipe' if smooth. 'Cog-wheel' tremor is movement like a ratchet; while there may be coexisting tremor which gives a feeling of cog-wheeling, true cog-wheeling is a form of rigidity independent of tremor.

◆ Rigidity is tested for by passively moving the limb through normal movements.

◆ Mild rigidity can be detected by 'activation', e.g. asking the patient to open and close the contra-lateral hand.

26 Rigidity. Neck tone is tested by flexion and extension (a). Leg tone is tested by flexion and extension at the knee and ankle (b). Arm tone is tested by flexion and extension at the elbow (c) and the wrist (d). During wrist examination, contra-lateral activation can increase tone, e.g. asking the patient to open and close the left hand while examining the right wrist may show an increase in tone, referred to as activated rigidity.

◆ Patients describe rigidity as muscle stiffness or sometimes pain. Occasionally, patients initially attend an orthopaedic department with a frozen shoulder, which is actually the first sign of PD. Pain in PD may also be caused by dystonia.

Tremor

- Definitions of tremor (**27**):
  - ◇ Tremor is an involuntary rhythmic oscillatory movement of a body part.
  - ◇ Rest tremor is typical of PD and occurs when the body part is relaxed, e.g. the arms and hands resting on the lap with the patient seated. Distraction may help 'bring out' a rest tremor, especially if the patient is anxious, e.g. asking the patient to count backwards.
  - ◇ Postural tremor occurs when a posture is sustained, e.g. an outstretched arm.
  - ◇ Action tremor occurs when performing a task, e.g. reaching for a cup.
- Tremor is the most widely known feature of PD.
- Tremor disappears during sleep.
- Tremor is the presenting symptom of PD in 40–70% of cases, and between 68% and 100% of PD patients will have rest tremor at some point during the course of their illness.

27 Tremor testing. Tremor is examined initially in the patient at rest, with the hands resting on the lap (a). If necessary a distraction technique, such as asking the patient to count backwards from 30, can help make the tremor more obvious. The patient is asked to elevate the arms (b). In Parkinson's disease, there is often a gap between the tremor present at rest, before a postural tremor is visible. This is called re-emergent tremor. The patient is asked to make a movement, such as the finger to nose test, to check for the presence of action tremor (c, d).

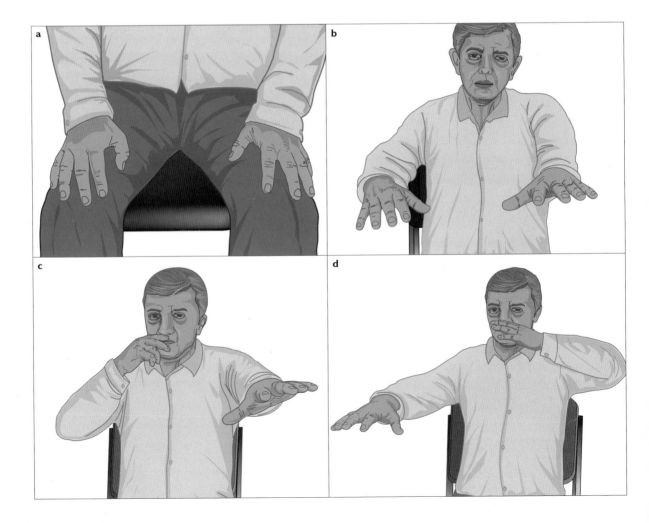

- 10–20% of PD patients do not have tremor.
- Classically tremor is at rest at a frequency of 4–6 Hz ('pill-rolling', as the tremor has a rotatory component), but the tremor can be at other frequencies.
- Tremor usually starts in one hand and arm, then progresses to the ipsilateral leg, later spreading contralaterally.
- Postural tremor is often present. There is latency between rest and postural tremor, meaning that the patient's arm and hand show rest tremor, which disappears (for about 9 s) when taking up a posture (e.g. holding up the arms), then the tremor re-emerges (hence sometimes called re-emergent tremor).
- Chin, jaw, and eyelid tremor can also occur in PD, but tremor of the whole head is rare.
  ◇ Head tremor, seen as nodding ('yes-yes' tremor) or shaking ('no-no' tremor), is a feature of ET or dystonic tremor rather than PD, but can rarely occur in PD.
- Worsening of tremor in PD prior to the next dose of medication indicates 'wearing-off' (patients may describe their tremor as worsening after they take a dose of medication, but this is usually because the dose has not yet taken effect, e.g. tremor which worsens in the first 20 minutes after taking a dose of levodopa is usually due to 'wearing off' rather than being a side-effect of the new dose).
- Tremor is often the most difficult symptom of the classic triad to treat. About half of cases will notice a treatment response with improvement in tremor, but tremor is seldom completely abolished. Patients are often troubled by the persistence of tremor despite therapy, and may report that the treatment is not working because tremor remains, even though bradykinesia has improved.
- Tremor of PD tends to increase with stress and anxiety, but this is not specific and is seen in many other types of tremor.
- Tremor dominance is a good prognostic feature.

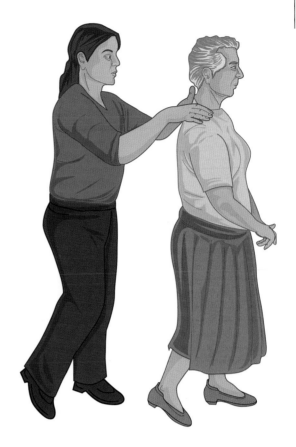

28 The pull test. This examines for postural instability. In health, the patient either remains upright without moving their legs in response to the test of retropulsion or steps back, but manages to maintain posture without difficulty. In PD there is initially a tendency to lose stability in this test and later the patient may simply fall backwards like a log, because the postural reflexes do not respond quickly enough – be prepared to catch the patient when doing this test!

Postural instability

- Patients report poor balance, unsteadiness, and falls.
- Postural instability is examined using the pull test (**28**). The examiner stands behind the patient and pulls back sharply on the patient's shoulders (the feet should be slightly apart, unlike their position in a Romberg's test). Patients may correct themselves in the early stages (retropulsion – the patient may take one or two steps back, but can correct themselves), but in advanced stages patients fall if unsupported.
- The severity of each of the cardinal features of PD can be scored numerically using the UPDRS for motor features (see Chapter 6).

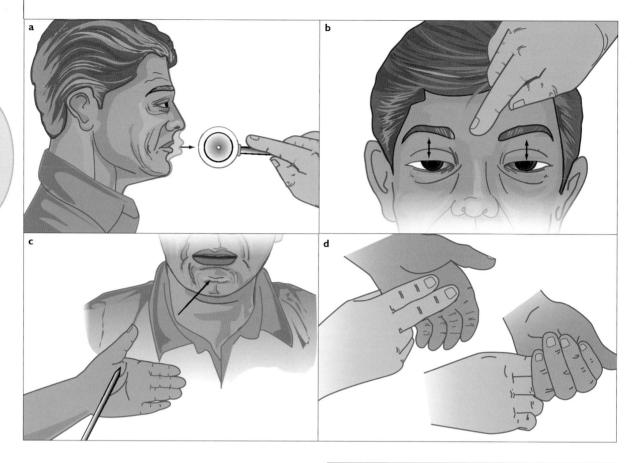

29 **Frontal lobe reflexes.** Pouting forwards of the lip (a); persistent blinking on tapping the forehead (b); chin twitch on quick scratch on the palm (palmomental reflex) (c); fingers flex on stroking the palm (d). These are not specific to PD but can help to support a diagnosis of a degenerative disorder compared to a benign condition such as ET.

30 **Clinical patterns in PD.** The presentation of PD varies: some patients have a tremor-dominant disorder while others are tremor negative, or have a greater predominance of the other components of the condition – referred to as akinetic–rigid cases.

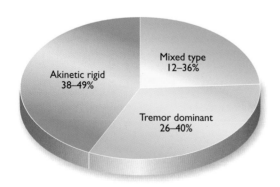

Frontal lobe reflexes

◆ These are usually present in PD but are not specific, as they occur in other brain disorders, such as MSA, PSP, stroke disease, and degenerative dementias. Frontal lobe refelexes are usually absent in healthy adults and in benign disorders such as ET. The palmomental reflex and glabellar tap are often positive from an early stage in PD, while the pout reflex and the grasp reflex are late features (**29**).

Subtypes of idiopathic PD

◆ Idiopathic PD can be subdivided into several variants (**30**):
  ◇ Tremor dominant (26–40% of cases).
  ◇ Akinetic–rigid (38–49% of cases).
  ◇ Mixed type (12–36% of cases).
◆ Different subtypes may have different rates of disease progression (tremor-dominant cases progress more slowly) and may represent a different underlying aetiology.

Problems in diagnosis

- Diagnostic certainty has been graded in different ways (e.g. by Calne *et al.* 1992) as follows (**31**):
  - ◇ Clinically possible (one of tremor, rigidity or bradykinesia, the tremor must be of recent onset, but may be resting or postural).
  - ◇ Clinically probable (any two of resting tremor, rigidity, bradykinesia, or impaired postural reflexes or alternatively asymmetric resting tremor, asymmetric rigidity or asymmetric bradykinesia are sufficient).
  - ◇ Clinically definite (any three of resting tremor, rigidity, bradykinesia or impairment of postural reflexes, alternatively any two of these features with one of the first three being asymmetrical).

31 Diagnostic criteria for PD according to Calne *et al.* (1992). These use the same cardinal features as the UK Brain Bank criteria and give added support to the diagnosis of PD in the presence of asymmetry.

- Gelb *et al.* (1999) proposed the following diagnostic criteria for PD.
- For a possible diagnosis of PD:
  - ◇ At least two of the following features are present, and at least one of these is brady-kinesia or tremor: resting tremor, brady-kinesia, rigidity, asymmetric onset (Group A).
  - *and*
  - ◇ *Either* none of the following features is present (Group B): postural instability in the first 3 years after symptom onset, freezing phenomena in the first 3 years, hallucinations unrelated to medications in the first 3 years, dementia preceding motor symptoms in the first year, supranuclear gaze palsy (other than restriction of upward gaze) or slowing or vertical saccades, severe symptomatic dys-autonomia unrelated to medications, docu-mentation of a condition known to produce parkinsonism and plausibly connected to the patient's symptoms (such as suitably located focal brain lesions or neuroleptic use within the past 6 months).

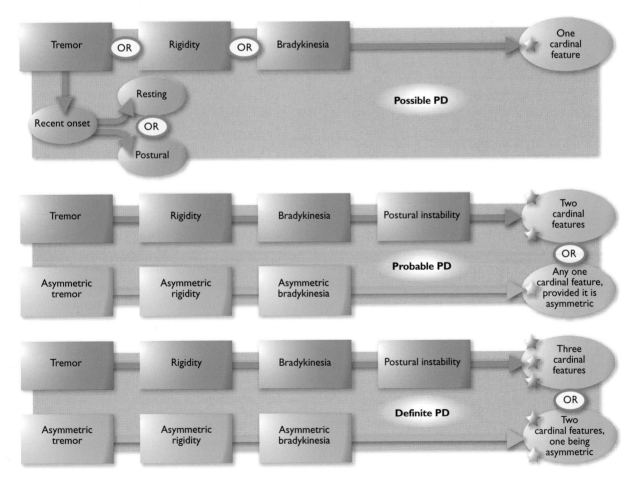

◇ *Or* symptoms have been present for less than 3 years, and none of the above features is present to date.

and

◇ *Either* substantial and sustained response to levodopa or a dopamine agonist (DA) has been documented.

◇ *Or* the patient has not had an adequate trial of levodopa or DA.

◆ A probable diagnosis of PD requires at least three of the four features of Group A *and* none of group B *and* a substantial and sustained response to levodopa or a DA.

◆ A definite diagnosis requires all the possible criteria *and* histopathological confirmation at autopsy.

Other similar presentations

Essential tremor

◆ In early disease the main differential from Parkinson's disease is ET.

◆ ET is approximately ten times more common than PD, with men and women eqully affected.

◆ The tremors of ET and PD are usually distinguished on clinical examination. Rest tremor is usually not present in ET. The tremor frequency of ET is similar to that of the latent postural tremor of PD, but can be faster (4–12 Hz). In ET, there is no latency on taking up a posture (i.e. the tremor starts as soon as a movement is initiated). The tremor of ET is generally in the plane of flexion/extension, whereas in PD there is also rotatory movement (e.g. at the wrist, hence the classic description of 'pill-rolling' tremor).

◆ In ET:

◇ Tremor is usually bilateral and occurs in posture and action tremor compared with the asymmetric rest tremor of PD.

◇ Family history is positive in approximately 50% of cases (AD mode of inheritance).

◇ Tremor improves with alcohol (the benefit of alcohol is more than merely the anxiolytic effect of alcohol).

◇ Tremor begins at a younger age (though the incidence of ET increases with age).

◇ Tremor is usually present for some time (often years), progresses considerably more slowly than PD, and is not associated with other parkinsonian features.

◇ Tremor of the head and neck is common in ET, whereas in PD head tremor is rare but chin and lip tremor do occur.

◆ In idiopathic PD tremor is usually asymmetrical, starts unilaterally, and occurs at rest, a positive family history is much less likely, the tremor does not generally respond to alcohol and other PD features (rigidity and bradykinesia) are present and the symptoms are usually more rapidly progressive.

◆ ET may not need pharmacological treatment, and an accurate diagnosis and reassurance are sometimes sufficient. In moderate to severe cases, beta-blockers may improve the tremor. If beta-blockers are ineffective, contraindicated or cause adverse effects, primidone can be tried alone or in combination (but can cause sedation and behavioural effects). Other treatments such as gabapentin and topiramate have some clinical trial evidence of benefit (although only small numbers of topiramate-treated cases completed the study). In severe intractable cases surgery such as thalamotomy or deep brain surgery should be considered.

Dystonic tremor

◆ Often associated with focal dystonia (e.g. torticollis – neck rotation due to dystonic spasm of the neck muscles).

◆ Postural tremor in the outstretched arms is typical, but there is often a rest component to arm tremor, and head, jaw, and leg tremor are also found in some cases.

◆ May be accompanied by parkinsonian features (e.g. facial hypomimia, reduced arm swing when walking).

◆ Clues to dystonia as a cause of tremor/parkinsonism include:

◇ Involuntary finger and/or thumb extension (or other dystonic posturing), noted for example during assessment of hand and arm movements such as lifting a cup.

◇ Head tilt from neck dystonia, e.g. torticollis (overactive sternomastoid, head rotation to opposite side), anterocollis (neck flexion), retrocollis (head pulled back, neck extension).

◇ Irregularity of limb tremor, which may occur in 'bursts', and worsening of tremor during tasks such as writing.

◇ Prior history of neck problems with an episode of self-remitting dystonia (e.g. 'wry neck' or torticollis).

Drug-induced parkinsonism

◆ In epidemiological studies between a third and a half of parkinsonism is caused by medication.

◆ Drug-induced parkinsonism (**32**) is sometimes difficult to distinguish from idiopathic PD, but certain features are helpful and, of course, the drug history is crucial.

◆ Although symptoms may be asymmetrical, a symmetrical presentation can be a hint to the presence of drug-induced parkinsonism.

◆ Neuroleptics are most commonly implicated (the newer atypical neuroleptics are less likely to induce parkinsonism, but still often cause milder forms of parkinsonism). In one prevalence study, 62% of patients on neuroleptics developed movement disorders, encompassing a mix of akathisia (31%), parkinsonism (23%), and tardive dyskinesia (32%).

◆ Anti-nausea agents (e.g. prochlorperazine, metoclopramide, cinnarizine) are other common culprits.

◆ Sodium valproate and tetrabenazine cause parkinsonism but at lower rates. Sodium valproate can also cause high-frequency tremor. Antidepressants and calcium antagonists have been implicated largely through case reports but data are not robust. As depression is common in PD (see Chapter 5) antidepressants can often be helpful, and worsening parkinsonism is seldom an issue in clinical practice.

◆ Although the parkinsonism usually improves on withdrawal of the offending drug, this may take many months and sometimes symptoms persist. If they persist, and especially if they worsen, for around 6 months or more after drug withdrawal, PD may have been unmasked (i.e. induced earlier than if the offending drug had not been prescribed) (**33**).

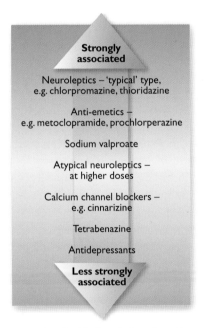

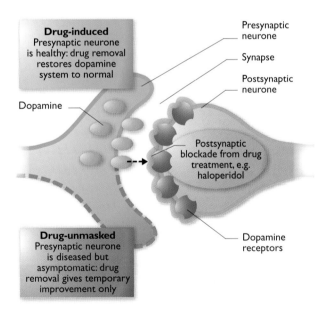

32 Drugs associated with drug-induced parkinsonism.
In general, traditional neuroleptics and anti-emetics should be avoided in PD, although there are some situations where behavioural disturbance or severe vomiting would justify their use. Strongly associated drugs have clear chemical mechanisms and more frequently cause parkinsonism (e.g. dopamine antagonists). Many individual drugs (not listed) have been reported to worsen parkinsonian symptoms but are of doubtful significance when considering the fluctuations inherent in PD.

33 Drug-induced versus drug-unmasked parkinsonism.
Drugs such as antipsychotics produce a blockade of post-synaptic dopamine receptors. Removal of the offending drug will return the patient to normal, although this can take weeks or months, with some evidence of residual parkinsonism in some patients even at 1 year. In some patients in the early pre-clinical stages of PD, features of early PD can be unmasked by the offending drug: the parkinsonism will improve initially but then deteriorate again when the drug is stopped.

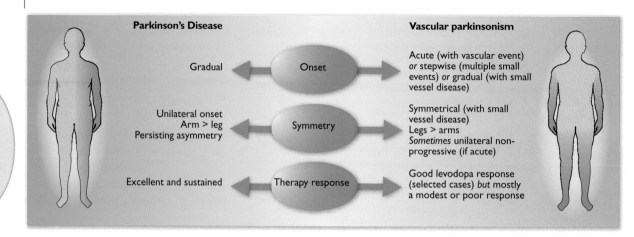

Parkinson's Disease		Vascular parkinsonism
Gradual	**Onset**	Acute (with vascular event) *or* stepwise (multiple small events) *or* gradual (with small vessel disease)
Unilateral onset Arm > leg Persisting asymmetry	**Symmetry**	Symmetrical (with small vessel disease) Legs > arms *Sometimes* unilateral non-progressive (if acute)
Excellent and sustained	**Therapy response**	Good levodopa response (selected cases) *but* mostly a modest or poor response

- Drug-unmasked PD can be distinguished from pure drug-induced parkinsonism using presynaptic functional dopamine imaging (PET or single photon emission computed tomography [SPECT]), which is abnormal in PD but normal in drug-induced parkinsonism. Most cases of drug-induced parkinsonism that persist represent unmasked PD.

Vascular parkinsonism

- Vascular parkinsonism (**34**) accounts for between 4.4% and 12% of all cases of parkinsonism, but a rate of 3–6% emerges if only studies using imaging or pathological diagnostic data are included.
- Incidence and prevalence of vascular parkinsonism increase with age and it is commoner in men than in women.
- The pattern is more typically of lower body involvement (while in idiopathic PD the arms and upper body are more affected). However, the upper body can be involved. Patients with vascular parkinsonism are more likely to be older, have postural instability, a history of falling, dementia, corticospinal findings, and incontinence.
- The original description by Critchley in the 1920s was of a predominant gait disorder (short steps – *marche à petit pas*) with additional features of dementia and pyramidal signs. Classically the presentation was described as an acute onset, which was symmetrical, without tremor, but with postural instability and a poor response to dopamine replacement therapy. However, the onset is much more typically insidious. In one series only about a quarter of cases of vascular

34 PD versus vascular parkinsonism. Distinguishing features are illustrated. The disorders may coexist, especially in the elderly patient.

parkinsonism were considered to have an acute onset with a new ischaemic stroke event – but even here the new event may have 'unmasked' an insidious process.

- There is therefore some suggestion that there may be two types of vascular parkinsonism:
  - ◇ With acute onset possibly associated with basal ganglia infarction.
  - ◇ With a more insidious onset, possibly associated with more diffuse subcortical white matter ischaemia.
- Vascular risk factors, including hypertension and diabetes, increase the risk of developing vascular parkinsonism. Other common vascular risk factors, including a family history of vascular disease, other evidence of vascular disease (ischaemic heart disease or peripheral vascular disease), hypercholesterolaemia, and smoking would seem likely to increase the risk of vascular parkinsonism, but evidence is lacking. A history of stroke is also a risk factor.
- Structural imaging may show basal ganglia infarcts, subcortical ischaemia or more diffuse small vessel changes. These findings support the diagnosis of vascular parkinsonism, but can of course also be present in the absence of clinical parkinsonism.
- In one series about 10% of cases with a basal ganglia stroke went on to develop vascular parkinsonism, but in another study 38% of patients with lacunar basal ganglia infarcts on MRI had clinical features of parkinsonism.

- Functional imaging, using SPECT or PET to check the integrity of presynaptic neurones, is abnormal in idiopathic PD, but normal in vascular parkinsonism (unless there is focal basal ganglia infarction).
- There are three pathological patterns of vascular parkinsonism:
    - Multiple lacunar infarcts clinically associated with gait disorder, pyramidal deficits, cognitive impairment, and pseudobulbar palsy.
    - Subcortical arteriosclerotic encephalopathy (Binswanger's disease) clinically associated with a progressive gait disorder and dementia.
    - Basal ganglia infarct (usually lacunar) – this type is rare.
- Idiopathic PD and vascular parkinsonism are relatively common in an ageing population and can coexist.
- Addressing vascular risk – control of hypertension, diabetes, hypercholesterolaemia, considering anti-platelet therapy and advising smoking cessation – seems sensible, although these therapeutic strategies have not been studied in vascular parkinsonism.
- Traditionally there is a poor therapeutic response to levodopa in vascular parkinsonism, but some evidence of a levodopa response in patients with pathological confirmation of vascular parkinsonism was noted in a case review (12 out of 17 patients had a good or excellent response documented). In clinical practice it is often appropriate to trial levodopa at a sufficient dose (where tolerated), and continue treatment if there is clinical benefit, but discontinue it after a reasonable length of time (3 months) if there is no response or adverse effects outweigh any benefit.

Multiple system atrophy

- MSA is clinically a combination of parkinsonism, autonomic dysfunction, and cerebellar features (**35**). The age-adjusted prevalence of MSA is about 4 per 100,000.
- Parkinsonism:
    - Bradykinesia, rigidity, postural instability, and tremor. In the consensus statement for the diagnosis of MSA, bradykinesia plus one of rigidity, postural instability or tremor are required to meet diagnostic criteria.

- Tremor is present in two thirds of patients with MSA. Less than 10% have the pill-rolling rest tremor which is typical of idiopathic PD. The tremor of MSA is usually of an irregular jerky type, noted during both posture and action and may be due to myoclonic jerks, which are sometimes touch or stretch sensitive.
- Autonomic problems:
    - Falls (relating to orthostatic hypotension, a fall in blood pressure of >20 mmHg systolic and >10 mmHg diastolic within 3 minutes of standing or head-up tilt, and low resting blood pressure).
    - Impotence.
    - Bladder instability (urinary incontinence or incomplete bladder emptying).
- Cerebellar signs:
    - Gait ataxia.
    - Speech problems (ataxic dysarthria).
    - Nystagmus (though this is not common).
    - Incoordination.
- Pyramidal signs can also occur:
    - Brisk reflexes.
    - Upgoing (extensor) plantar reflexes.

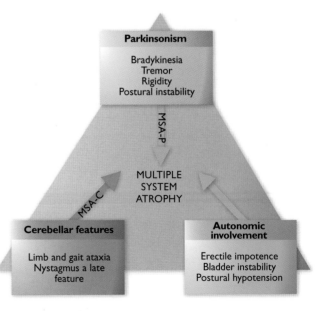

35 The components of MSA. Patients may present with features from one of the components initially but ultimately the features from the remaining system degenerations will emerge. MSA-C = multiple system atrophy (cerebellar); MSA-P = multiple system atrophy (parkinsonism).

- Patients with a predominantly parkinsonian presentation are classified as having the MSA-P subtype of MSA (formerly known as striatonigral degeneration); those with stronger cerebellar features are labelled as subtype MSA-C (formerly sporadic olivopontocerebellar atrophy).
- MSA-P is between two and four times commoner than MSA-C.
- Glial cytoplasmic inclusions (GCIs) are the pathological hallmark of MSA. GCIs display alpha-synuclein immunoreactivity.
- The mean age of onset is 54 years (younger than idiopathic PD), and there are no known pathologically proven cases with symptoms developing before the age of 30 years.
- Dyskinesia can develop, especially orofacial.
- Dementia is uncommon. In the consensus diagnostic categories and exclusion criteria for MSA, the Diagnostic and Statistical Manual (DSM) criteria for dementia are considered exclusion criteria for MSA. However, alterations of personality and mood can occur.

Progressive supranuclear palsy
- The median age of onset is 60–65 years.
- The median disease duration from diagnosis to death varies between 5.9 years and 9.7 years.
- The age-adjusted prevalence is about 6 per 100,000.

- Parkinsonism occurs, particularly axial rigidity (hence neck and trunk movements are more affected than limbs) plus:
  - ◇ Early falls (with a tendency to fall backwards, 'like a tree trunk').
  - ◇ Loss of vertical eye movement (unable to look up or down on command but able to follow a moving target in early stages) (**36**); but there have been pathologically confirmed cases without gaze paresis, so it is not a universal finding.
  - ◇ Speech and swallowing difficulty.
  - ◇ Dementia.
  - ◇ Upper motor neurone signs.
- Neurofibrillary tangles and neuropil threads in the basal ganglia and other parts of the brainstem and Tau positive tufts are the pathological features.

36 Gaze paresis in PSP. The patient is unable to look down (a) or up (b) voluntarily, but there is some ability for the eyes to move upwards (relative to head position) when the neck is flexed (c) – this is called the oculocephalic manoeuvre (but it may be difficult to perform because of neck rigidity, which is another key feature of the condition).

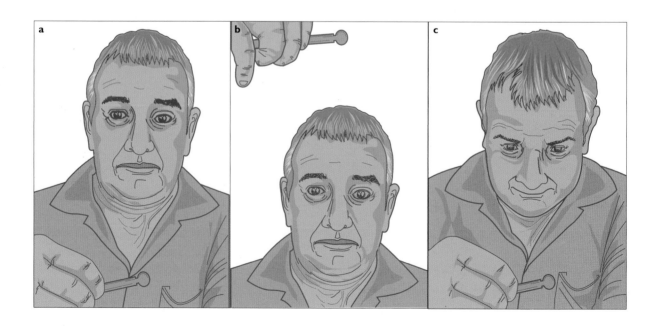

Corticobasal degeneration

- Parkinsonism occurs along with cortical dysfunction.
- Parkinsonism manifests as an akinetic rigid syndrome which is unresponsive to levodopa.
- Cognitive impairment is a dominant feature.
- Symptoms usually start after the age of 60.
- Unilateral bradykinesia and rigidity occur with or without tremor.
- An irregular jerky arm is typical.
- Progressive gait disturbance, dystonia, dysphagia, and dysarthria may occur.
- Features include apraxia (patients complain that their limb does not understand tasks), cortical sensory loss, and memory loss.
- Other signs include: myoclonus, corticospinal signs, choreoathetosis, supranuclear gaze abnormalities, and blepharospasm.
- Symptoms spread contralaterally within 1 year.
- Patients may have an 'alien' limb, e.g. if they are scratching, they deny that it is their own hand (a feature that everyone remembers but not all patients develop).
- The cause is unknown, but there is an accumulation of the Tau protein.
- Structural neuroimaging shows cortical atrophy, and functional neuroimaging shows reduced cortical blood flow in the fronto-parieto-temporal area which is sometimes asymmetrical.
- There is no specific treatment, and supportive multidisciplinary care is required.
- Pharmacotherapy may include antidepressants and a trial of dopaminergic therapy. Clonazepam may help myoclonus, and baclofen can be used for muscle spasm.

Wilson's disease

- A genetic (autosomal recessive) disorder with a deficiency of a copper-carrier membrane protein.
- The abnormal gene is located on chromosome 13.
- Should be considered in all young (<50 years) patients presenting with parkinsonism.
- 50% of patients present with neurological or psychiatric symptoms, and the remainder present with symptoms of liver disease, usually in childhood (but up to age 53).
- Serum caeruloplasmin is low and urinary copper is raised.

- Kayser-Fleischer rings (a brown deposit in the cornea, around the outer edge of the iris which represents a deposition of copper in Descement's membrane):
  - ◇ May be seen by naked eye especially in patients with blue irises.
  - ◇ Usually require an ophthalmological slit lamp examination.
- Treatment is with penicillamine or other copper-chelating agents.

Dementia with Lewy bodies

- DLB accounts for about 20% of all dementia.
- May present as a predominant dementia with some extrapyramidal signs, or initially as parkinsonism with early-onset dementia. The term Parkinson's disease with dementia (PDD) has been used when parkinsonism predates the development of dementia by at least one year, and DLB when dementia starts before that (**37**).
- Visual hallucinations, delusions, and psychosis may occur in the absence of dopaminergic therapy.
- Cognitive decline is progressive but may fluctuate (there are lucid periods when mental performance is much nearer normal).

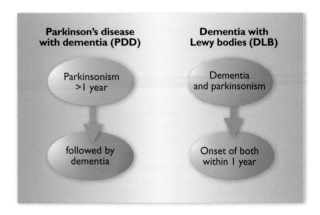

37 Differentiating PD dementia from dementia with Lewy bodies. This working definition is useful in clinical studies and in clinical care, but the disorders are likely to represent a continuum.

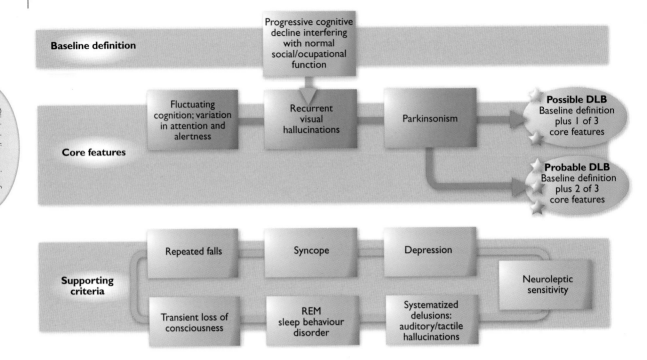

Baseline definition

Progressive cognitive decline interfering with normal social/ocupational function

Core features

Fluctuating cognition; variation in attention and alertness

Recurrent visual hallucinations

Parkinsonism

Possible DLB
Baseline definition plus 1 of 3 core features

Probable DLB
Baseline definition plus 2 of 3 core features

Supporting criteria

Repeated falls

Syncope

Depression

Neuroleptic sensitivity

Transient loss of consciousness

REM sleep behaviour disorder

Systematized delusions: auditory/tactile hallucinations

- The Scientific Issues Committee of the Movement Disorder society task force formed consensus criteria for the clinical diagnosis of DLB.
- To reach a *possible* diagnosis the inclusion criteria are (**38**):
  - Progressive cognitive decline of sufficient magnitude to interfere with normal social or occupational function (prominent or persistent memory impairment may not necessarily occur in the early stages but is usually evident with progression; deficits on tests of attention and frontal-subcortical skills and visuospatial ability may be especially prominent).
  - One of three core features: fluctuating cognition with pronounced variations in attention and alertness; recurrent visual hallucinations; parkinsonism.
- Supportive criteria are:
  - Repeated falls.
  - Syncope.
  - Transient loss of consciousness.
  - Neuroleptic sensitivity.
  - Systematized delusions, hallucinations in other modalities (e.g. hearing voices or feeling the touch of a visualized figure).
  - Depression.
  - Rapid eye movement (REM) sleep behaviour disorder (RBD).

38 DDLB diagnostic criteria. The diagnosis of possible or probable DLB depends on three core features and a range of supportive criteria.

- To reach a *probable* diagnosis of DLB patients need to fulfil the *possible* criteria plus one more core feature.
- Exclusion criteria for both *possible* and *probable* are stroke disease or evidence of any other brain disorder sufficient to account for the clinical picture.
- Autopsy is required to reach a definite diagnosis.
- Management often involves reduction and sometimes discontinuation of antiparkinson medication – particularly anticholinergics, selegiline, amantadine, and DAs. Patients are often sensitive to neuroleptics, which are usually avoided. Cognitive function may improve with cholinesterase inhibitors. DAs in conjunction with atypical neuroleptics have sometimes been used successfully.

Normal-pressure hydrocephalus

◆ This is a rare condition where parkinsonism may occur with normal-pressure hydrocephalus and primary empty sella.

◆ In addition to parkinsonism, symptoms are of urinary incontinence, gait disturbance, and dementia.

◆ It is distinguished from PD by:
  ◇ Rigidity, tremor, and bradykinesia tending to be less common than in PD.
  ◇ There being a limited if any response to levodopa.
  ◇ Incontinence is usually urinary, but may also be faecal.
  ◇ Dementia may progress less rapidly than in Alzheimer's or in PD dementia.

◆ Structural neuroimaging aids diagnosis.

◆ Surgical shunting should be considered. However, the risks of surgery may outweigh potential benefit, particularly when poor prognostic features, including dementia, long-standing symptoms, and cortical atrophy, are present.

◆ Normal-pressure hydrocephalus may be confused with PD or vascular dementia.

Red flags (alerts)

◆ An assessment for PD should check for 'red flags' suggesting an alternative diagnosis (**39**):
  ◇ Early falls – Parkinson-plus syndrome (usually PSP or MSA).
  ◇ Early dementia – DLB, PSP, corticobasal degeneration, Alzheimer's disease.
  ◇ Apraxia and alien limb – corticobasal degeneration.
  ◇ Early pronounced autonomic features (impotence, postural hypotension) – MSA.
  ◇ Sudden onset of symptoms – cerebrovascular event.
  ◇ No rest tremor.
  ◇ Symmetrical onset and signs.
  ◇ Predominance of axial symptoms.
  ◇ Poor therapy response.
  ◇ Rapid progression.
  ◇ Alzheimer's disease patients often have parkinsonian symptoms.

◆ These features raise the possibility of an alternative diagnosis, including other forms of degenerative parkinsonism, which can be collectively considered as the *Parkinson-plus* disorders (but note that Parkinson-plus is not a diagnosis in itself):
  ◇ MSA.
  ◇ PSP.

◆ Death usually occurs within 5–10 years (however these figures may be subject to referral bias and survival can be longer).

Red flags in the diagnosis of PD

PRESENCE OF	SUGGESTS
As an early feature:	
Falls	MSA or PSP
Dementia	Lewy body dementia, PSP, corticobasal degeneration, or Alzheimer's
Pronounced autonomic features	MSA
Sudden onset	Stroke
Apraxia, alien limb	Cortico-basal degeneration
Rapid progression	One of the Parkinson-plus disorders
Absence of rest tremor	Benign tremor disorder (essential tremor, dystonic tremor)

39 **Red flags.** The presence of one or more of these features suggests an alternative diagnosis.

Misdiagnosis

◆ Misdiagnosis is common.

◆ Diagnostic revision is 25–50% in community studies.

◆ Lower misdiagnosis rates (10–25%) occur in specialist centres, though this is based on diagnosis made later in the course of the disease (i.e. the last antemortem visit diagnosis compared against autopsy results is likely to reveal more accurate clinical diagnosis compared against the initial diagnosis at presentation).

◆ It may take time for the diagnosis to emerge.

◆ PD is sometimes mistaken for primary depression (reduced facial expression, motor slowing, constipation), hypothyroidism or slowing due to normal ageing.

◆ Striatal toe – a cramp or muscle spasm in the forefoot, in which the great toe involuntary extends (dorsiflexes, i.e. points upwards) is sometimes the first sign of PD. Striatal toe is a form of dystonia, and when dystonia is the presenting feature of PD, the feet are involved in the vast majority of cases.

◆ Frozen shoulder – unilateral frozen shoulder resulting from rigidity and bradykinesia – is sometimes a presenting feature.

◆ Psychogenic movement disorder – early-onset PD, especially with any atypical features, is sometimes mislabelled as psychogenic.

◆ Psychogenic parkinsonism is rare. Suggestive features include abrupt onset, rapid initial progression which plateaus, bizarre gait, exaggerated slowness, and psychological overlay. The levodopa response varies between nil and excellent, but drug-induced motor complications and advancing complications (such as dementia) do not occur. Functional presynaptic dopamine imaging can help differentiate psychogenic parkinsonism (normal scan) from idiopathic PD (abnormal scan). Psychological complications occur in PD, and some manifest physically such as tremor, hyperventilation, and other involuntary movements.

CHAPTER 3

Diagnostic testing and neuroimaging

Dopaminergic challenge tests

◆ Levodopa and apomorphine challenge tests may help to determine whether a patient is responsive to dopaminergic therapy (**40**).

◆ Levodopa challenge: score the patient before and 60 min after a single high dose of levodopa (e.g. 250 mg). (Levodopa is given in the usual way in conjunction with a dopa-decarboxylase inhibitor, as Sinemet (co-careldopa) or Madopar (co-beneldopa), in a standard-release formulation).

◆ Apomorphine challenge: score the patient before and 20 minutes after sequential doses of sub-cutaneous apomorphine (e.g. 1 mg, 3 mg, 5 mg, but stopping once benefit or side-effects emerge).

40 Dopaminergic challenge testing. Motor score responses to dopaminergic challenge tests – apomorphine and single high-dose levodopa – are shown.

◆ Pretreatment with an antinauseant (e.g. domperi-done) reduces nausea and hypotension side-effects, and this is especially important for apomorphine. Pretreatment is less important when testing a patient who is already taking antiparkinson medication, as they have more tolerance to side-effects (challenge testing in this situation is to check an uncertain therapy response).

◆ A positive response is declared when the reduction in motor score is 20% or more (sometimes a target of 30% is set). Low pretreat-ment scores in early PD (due to mild clinical features) make determination of improvement difficult so that challenge testing is better avoided when the baseline motor score is less than 10. Other parameters have been used, e.g. walking speed.

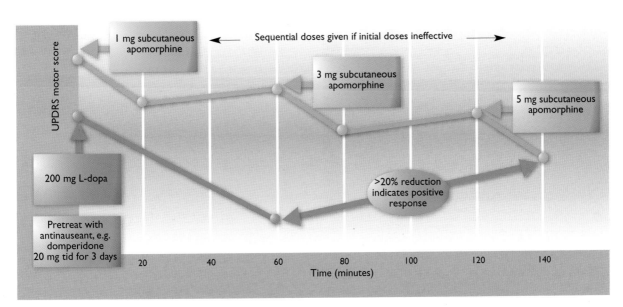

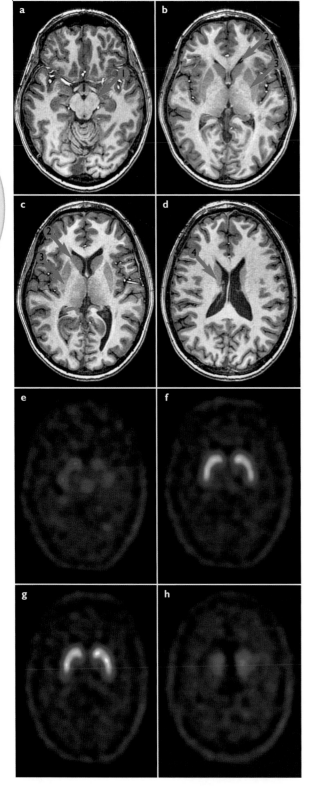

◆ Some patients do not show a response to a challenge test but do show a response to longer-term oral therapy. For this reason, challenge tests cannot be used to declare a patient unresponsive to dopaminergic medication.

◆ Challenge tests have a limited role in routine clinical practice, but may be part of a research protocol. They are occasionally helpful in a diagnostically difficult patient. If a challenge test is planned in a patient who has yet to start treatment, and in whom the initial oral treatment choice would be a dopamine agonist (DA) rather than levodopa, then apomorphine is the preferred challenge test. This is because levodopa may 'prime' the patient for the earlier development of dyskinesia.

◆ Assessing the response to apomorphine is part of initiating this treatment, for intermittent use for sudden 'off' periods (see Chapter 8).

Olfactory testing

◆ Olfaction (sense of smell) is impaired in PD (see Chapter 2).

◆ Smell testing is best performed using standardized methods, e.g. University of Pennsylvania Smell Identification Test (UPSIT) or Sniffin' sticks.

◆ Impaired olfaction correlates with functional neuroimaging abnormalities in early PD.

◆ Twin studies suggest that olfactory abnormalities occur <7 years before the onset of PD.

Structural neuroimaging

◆ The basal ganglia and substantia nigra are well visualized on MRI and can be matched to areas of dopamine activity on functional imaging (**41**).

◆ Although structural imaging is quite often performed in patients with suspected idiopathic PD, it is usually normal, and may therefore be reserved for patients more likely to show abnormalities.

41 Dopamine activity. MRI scanning at the level of the brainstem (a) and through the caudate and putamen (b–d); matching FP-CIT SPECT dopamine transporter activity (e–h). There is some activity at the substantia nigra level (e) but the greatest activity is through the middle of the striatum (f–g). *Figures courtesy of Dr Jim Patterson, Glasgow.*

I	Substantia nigra	2	Head of caudate
3	Putamen	4	Body of caudate

- Incidental abnormalities may be seen, such as basal ganglia calcification (**42**).
- Structural neuroimaging may assist in diagnosis in some patients with dual pathology, e.g. PD plus cerebrovascular disease (suggested clinically, for example, by prominence of walking and balance problems).

- Structural neuroimaging may be indicated if:
  - Tremor is acute in onset (suggesting a vascular cause).
  - Features remain unilateral (since PD should become bilateral).
  - There are features unusual for PD (e.g. early gait ataxia, incontinence, or frontal features suggesting hydrocephalus).
  - Lower-body involvement is prominent (especially with vascular disease at other body sites or risk factors for vascular disease, e.g. hypertension).
  - There is a poor response to antiparkinson therapy (in association with some of the above features).
- Structural neuroimaging may show localized abnormalities on MRI in cases of degenerative parkinsonism other than idiopathic PD (although none of these techniques reliably distinguishes Parkinson-plus from PD at an early stage), e.g.:
  - Midbrain atrophy in MSA (which sometimes results in a brainstem appearance called the 'hot cross bun' sign) (**43**).
  - A hyperintense putaminal rim in MSA (this may be seen in normal patients using high-field (3-Tesla) scanning, but is absent on the fluid-attenuated inversion recovery (FLAIR) sequence).

Diagnostic testing and neuroimaging

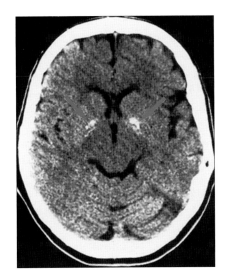

42 Basal ganglia calcification. This was an incidental finding in a patient with idiopathic PD.

43 Posterior fossa atrophy and the 'hot cross bun' sign. Normal brainstem and basal cistern size (a). Increase in basal cistern size (circled area) in a patient with MSA (b). In another patient with MSA (c), brainstem atrophy gives a distinctive appearance, referred to as the 'hot cross bun' sign, based on a traditional English bun appearance (inset).

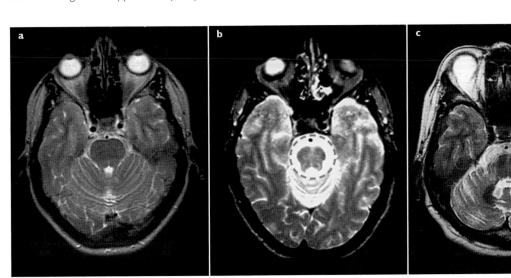

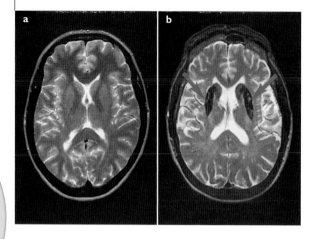

44 MRI scans showing Hallevorden–Spatz disease.
Increased iron deposition in the putamen in a case of pantothenate kinase-associated neurodegeneration (also called
Hallervorden–Spatz disease and sometimes referred to as
neurodegeneration with brain iron accumulation). The scan on
the left (a) shows normal basal ganglia structures and appearance. The scan on the right (b) shows increased signal bilaterally in the putamen (arrows) caused by iron deposition.

◇ Morphometric changes in Wilson's disease
(i.e. reductions from normal in the diameter
and other measurements of brainstem size).

◇ Abnormal iron deposition in the putamen
(**44**) in the rare syndrome of pantothenate
kinase-associated neurodegeneration
(Hallevorden–Spatz disease).

Structural brain causes of parkinsonism

◆ Cerebrovascular disease:

◇ Ischaemic changes in a periventricular
pattern (subcortical white matter), relating to
small vessel disease (e.g. hypertension,
diabetes) (**45**).

◇ Diffuse cerebral white matter lesions mainly
frontally are reported in one series.

◇ Small basal ganglia infarcts may cause acute
onset tremor or parkinsonism; cases of sub-
clinical PD might be unmasked by acute
ischaemic damage.

◇ The classical clinical pattern of lower-body
parkinsonism has been attributed to
ischaemic disruption of pathways between
primary and supplementary motor cortex and
the basal ganglia and cerebellum.

◇ Diffuse white matter lesions may initially
cause an isolated gait disorder without other
parkinsonian features.

45 MRI scan showing cerebrovascular disease. There is
evidence of small vessel cerebrovascular disease at multiple
sites, including the typical periventricular location (a, b,
arrowed). FP-CIT SPECT was nomal (c) and the patient's
parkinsonism, which was principally axial and lower body,
showed a poor response to levodopa.

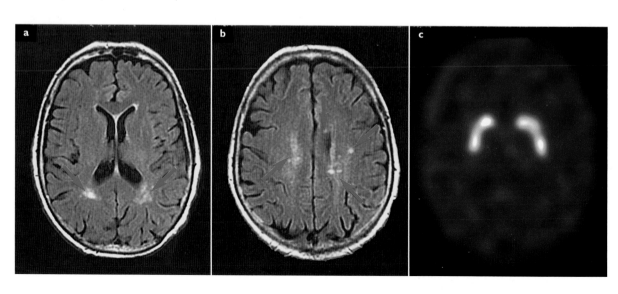

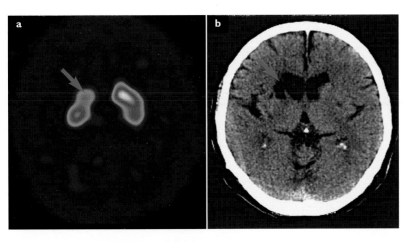

46 Focal basal ganglia abnormalities. FP-CIT SPECT (a) showing reduced caudate dopamine activity (arrow) and matching CT brain (b) showing infarction in the caudate at the same site. The patient did not have any clinical features of tremor or parkinsonism.
Figure courtesy of Dr Jim Patterson, Glasgow.

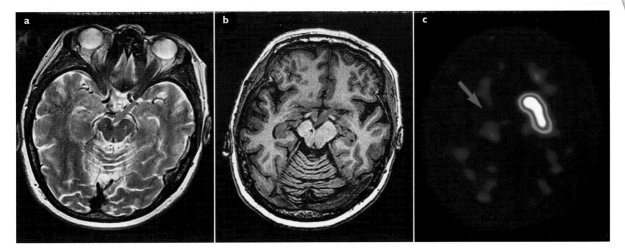

47 Damage to the substantia nigra. MRI showing unilateral vascular lesion (prior haemorrhage) in the substantia nigra (arrowed, a, b). The patient had left-sided tremor and parkinsonism, which responded to levodopa. Presynaptic dopamine activity was absent (c, arrow), while postsynaptic activity was increased through upregulation (not shown).
Figure courtesy of Dr Jim Patterson, Glasgow.

◇ As well as causing lower-body parkinsonism, vascular damage may cause a clinical picture very like idiopathic PD, PSP, or corticobasal degeneration.

◇ Vascular lesions may cause focal basal ganglia abnormalities without causing parkinsonism (**46**).

◇ Lesions within the substantia nigra, or affecting the nigrostriatal pathway, can affect dopamine activity within the striatum, resulting in parkinsonism (**47**).

◆ Arteriovenous malformation or cavernoma (**48**), typically in basal ganglia.

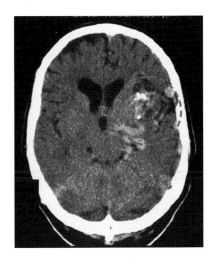

48 Arteriovenous malformation. Left-sided arteriovenous malformation (circled) in a patient presenting with clinical features suggesting early right-sided hemiparkinsonism. The patient was managed conservatively and did not progress to bilateral involvement.

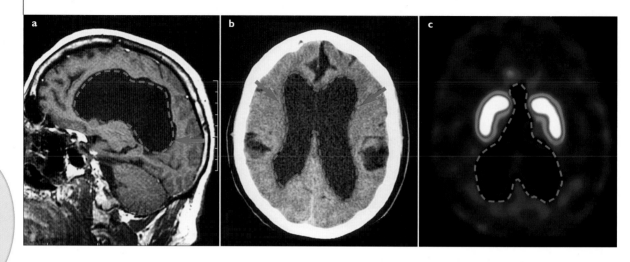

49 Hydrocephalus. This patient had parkinsonism with predominant gait ataxia. Ventricular enlargement is obvious both on MRI (a) and CT (b). FP-CIT SPECT showed normal dopamine activity (c) but also gave a hint of the hydrocephalus (dotted area with absence of even background tracer uptake). The patient improved on ventricular decompression.
FP-CIT scan courtesy of Dr Jim Patterson, Glasgow.

- Hydrocephalus (**49**):
  ◇ Obstructive (relieved by ventriculostomy or drainage).
  ◇ Normal-pressure hydrocephalus – enlarged ventricles disproportionate to any cortical atrophy.

Functional neuroimaging

- PET and SPECT can identify pre- and post-synaptic components of the dopaminergic system in PD and other types of degenerative parkinsonism (**50, 51**).
- There is some geographical variation in availability of these tests.
- The cost of such scans may not be reimbursed in healthcare schemes.
- Such testing is not required for uncomplicated cases with typical features.
- Research evaluation of other systems is of interest:
  ◇ Serotonin (5-hydroxytryptamine or 5-HT) in relation to tremor.
  ◇ Cholinergic systems in relation to dementia.

Mechanisms in functional neuroimaging

- ^{18}F-dopa (or ^{18}-fluoro-dopa):
  ◇ Is a marker of presynaptic dopamine activity.
  ◇ Is taken up in the presynaptic neurone and converted to ^{18}F-dopamine by decarboxylation.
  ◇ Requires omission of antiparkinson medication before the scan (for 12 hours).
  ◇ Underestimates the true degree of dopaminergic loss, due to upregulation (i.e. increased turnover within the presynaptic neurone, to compensate for dopamine deficiency).
- Dopamine transporter ligands. Several isotopes function as markers of dopamine transporter activity (i.e. re-uptake of dopamine from the synaptic cleft into the presynaptic neurone) (**50b**).
  ◇ Dopamine transporter studies overestimate the true degree of dopaminergic loss, due to downregulation (i.e. less dopamine transporter activity than normal, to preserve active dopamine in the synaptic cleft).
- Dopamine transporter ligands are cocaine analogues but do not have psychotropic effects:
  ◇ FP-CIT (DaTSCAN, GE Healthcare) is licensed in Europe to aid diagnosis in cases of clinical uncertainty between benign tremor disorders and PD.
  ◇ Beta-CIT, IPT, and TRODAT-1 are similar ligands used mainly in research.
- FP-CIT, Beta-CIT, IPT and TRODAT-1 are all used primarily in SPECT studies; studies of the dopamine transporter with PET have used, e.g. ^{18}F-CFT and ^{11}C-WIN.

- Uptake in regions of interest is usually compared to a reference area such as the cerebellum to calculate an uptake ratio (for SPECT studies; in PET there is no need to calculate a ratio to a reference range as absolute values are measured).
- Direct comparisons between studies using different ligands, or using different scanning equipment, are difficult; typical normal uptake ratios of 2.3 for FP-CIT compare to 5.5 for Beta-CIT and 2 for TRODAT.
- Test–retest reliability affects interpretation of repeat scans in individual patients:
  - ◇ It is 7% for FP-CIT in normal subjects and PD patients.
  - ◇ It is between 13 and 17% for Beta-CIT.

- There is no requirement to stop levodopa, DA, or monoamine oxidase B inhibitor (MAOB-I) therapy before presynaptic SPECT scanning.
  - ◇ Interaction studies show negligible if any effect on scan results comparing drug-naïve patients at baseline to patients on anti-parkinson therapy for up to 10 weeks.
  - ◇ Repeat scanning after drug withdrawal also shows no effect of short-term drug treatment on presynaptic activity (levodopa up to 750 mg, selegiline 10 mg, Beta-CIT study).
- Amphetamine and sympathomimetic agents should be stopped 4 weeks before scanning; some such agents are present in nasal decongestants.

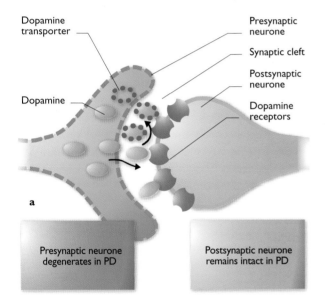

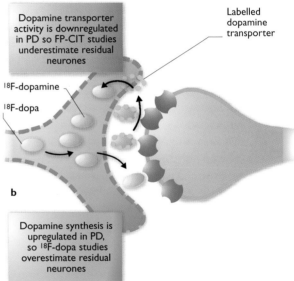

50 PET and SPECT in PD. Dopamine is synthesized in the presynaptic neurone and released into the synaptic cleft, with extracellular dopamine being reabsorbed via transporter proteins (a). ^{18}F-dopa is a PET marker for dopamine synthesis, while dopamine transporters are isotope-labelled by FP-CIT, Beta-CIT, TRODAT, etc., to trace activity (b). Although there is evidence of compensatory mechanisms, such effects are minor relative to the loss of neurones even in early PD.

Presynaptic neurone	Postsynaptic neurone
● Degenerates in idiopathic PD	● Available for antiparkinson therapy benefit
● Degenerates in Parkinson-plus disorders	● Pre- and post-synaptic degeneration = limited therapy benefit in Parkinson-plus disorders
● Site of metabolism of levodopa	● Blockade by anti-psychotics/anti-emetics may unmask early PD or cause reversible parkinsonism
● Turnover of levodopa and dopamine is regulated in PD	● Dopamine agonists act at various receptor sites

51 Neurone abnormalities. Differentiating features increase synaptic versus postsynaptic dopamine neurones in parkinsonism. The characteristics of abnormalities occurring in the pre-synaptic and postsynaptic neurones in PD and Parkinson-plus disorders as well as drug effects are shown.

Presynaptic dopamine imaging as a diagnostic and research tool in PD

◆ Imaging findings need to be considered separately for:
  ◇ Patients presenting with possible PD (i.e. already symptomatic), who may later have repeat scans (in research studies).
  ◇ Relatives of patients with PD, who may be identified as having early (preclinical) PD.

Patients presenting with possible PD

◆ At first presentation with PD there is usually at least 30% reduction from normal in presynaptic dopamine activity on PET or SPECT.
  ◇ This is consistent with the degree of substantia nigra cell loss in early PD seen in postmortem studies.
◆ Initial changes are often bilateral but more marked in the putamen contralateral to symptom onset (suggesting 'presymptomatic' loss in the initially clinically unaffected side)(**52b**).
  ◇ Progressive loss occurs in putamen then caudate and eventually low activity is almost symmetrical (**52c**).
  ◇ PET studies of the dopamine transporter showed putamen reduction to 42% of normal controls, and caudate reduction to 76% of normal controls, at around 2 years' duration of symptoms.
  ◇ Presynaptic dopamine deficiency occurs in a number of other degenerative disorders which feature parkinsonism (**53**).

◆ The pattern of loss differs from normal ageing, where neuronal loss occurs evenly in different brain areas.
◆ Clinical severity of bradykinesia and rigidity correlates with presynaptic dopaminergic activity (but tremor severity does not correlate). There is an overall correlation of scan results with H&Y scoring of PD patients.
◆ Clinical severity in relation to the degree of dopaminergic loss is less in patients with the PARK 2 (Parkin) variant of PD, compared to other PD patients (**54**).

52 Presynaptic dopamine imaging.

(a) The comma-shaped caudate and putamen on FP-CIT SPECT (DaTSCAN) are shown. This pattern is seen in healthy individuals and patients with ET.

(b) A reduction in the left more than right putamen (arrow) but bilaterally abnormal with reduced caudate activity. This patient had 2 years' symptoms and greater clinical involvement on the right side of the body, matching the more marked putamen loss on the left side.

(c) An advanced case: virtually no activity in either putamen. Caudate activity is bilaterally reduced, particularly on the patient's right side (arrow). Some asymmetry may persist clinically throughout the patient's life and matches the dopamine levels seen on functional dopaminergic brain imaging.

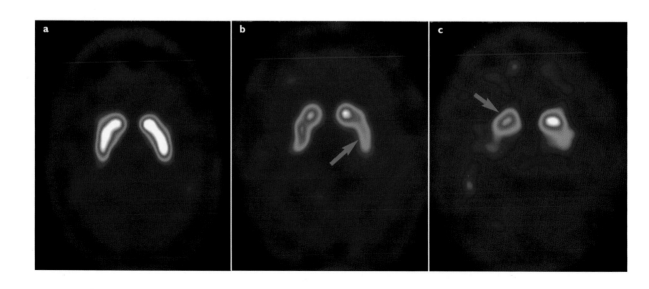

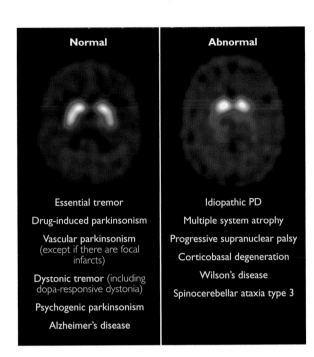

Normal	Abnormal
Essential tremor	Idiopathic PD
Drug-induced parkinsonism	Multiple system atrophy
Vascular parkinsonism (except if there are focal infarcts)	Progressive supranuclear palsy
	Corticobasal degeneration
Dystonic tremor (including dopa-responsive dystonia)	Wilson's disease
Psychogenic parkinsonism	Spinocerebellar ataxia type 3
Alzheimer's disease	

◆ Distinguishing idiopathic PD from MSA, PSP, and other forms of degenerative parkinsonism has proved difficult.

◇ Higher degrees of asymmetry in dopaminergic activity are more likely in PD than MSA or PSP (which matches the clinical pattern of asymmetry in these disorders, i.e. PD is more likely to present with asymmetry, and remain more troublesome for one body side than the other).

◇ Mapping techniques for scan readings offer the potential to distinguish these disorders, since striatal loss tends to be more uniform, for example, in MSA than in PD (the putamen:caudate ratio has been used in this setting but more sophisticated techniques are probably required).

53 Differentiating parkinsonian and tremor disorders. The left panel shows conditions in which normal presynaptic dopamine imaging occurs. The right panel shows conditions in which abnormal presynaptic dopamine imaging occurs.

54 Dopamine activity and the rate of change. There is evidence of a varying rate of dopamine loss as the disease progresses. Patients with parkin-positive PD show a somewhat different pattern to those with sporadic PD: younger age of onset, lower dopamine activity at presentation, but subsequently a slower decline. This is one source of variability in comparing clinical to imaging findings in PD.

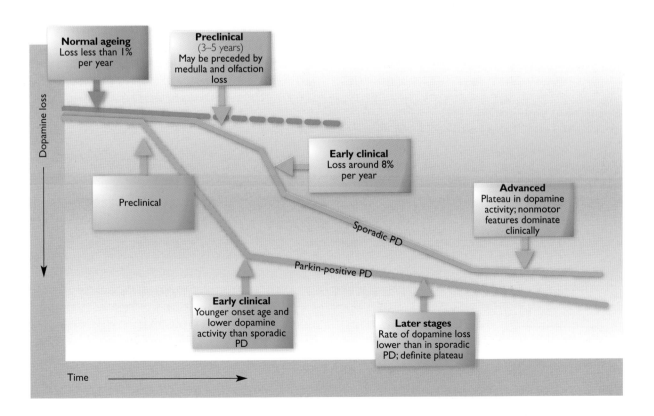

Normal ageing
Loss less than 1% per year

Preclinical (3–5 years)
May be preceded by medulla and olfaction loss

Dopamine loss

Preclinical

Early clinical
Loss around 8% per year

Advanced
Plateau in dopamine activity; nonmotor features dominate clinically

Sporadic PD

Parkin-positive PD

Early clinical
Younger onset age and lower dopamine activity than sporadic PD

Later stages
Rate of dopamine loss lower than in sporadic PD; definite plateau

Time

Progression rates in PD

◆ Annual loss occurs at around 8% (FP-CIT) and 6–11% (Beta-CIT) in PD (compared to an age-related change of 0.3–1% per annum).

◆ Annual progression at 4.7% (of normal mean) occurs on repeat ^{18}F-dopa PET studies (which suggests a 5-year duration for preclinical PD).

◇ The rate of putamen loss may be higher than that of caudate loss (more than double in one study) but differences arise from calculation techniques and study timings.

◆ The rate of change may be faster around the time of clinical presentation than later during the disease course.

◇ A 'reverse exponential' rate of loss may occur at disease onset.

◇ Later progression rates are more stable.

◇ Progression rates were steady for up to 7 years' disease duration when comparing scans at 0, 2, and 3 years (0 = study entry, not disease onset).

◇ Selection bias – including less severely affected patients in later studies – may influence these observations.

◆ The test–retest variability of these techniques indicates that progression rates are not reliable for individual patients, but require group studies.

◆ Continued dopaminergic loss has been shown to occur after subthalamic stimulation (^{18}F-dopa PET study in 30 patients before and 16 months after deep brain surgery; conducted to determine whether such surgery might be neuroprotective).

Relatives of patients with PD

◆ Heterozygotes for Parkin (which is related to the PARK2 genetic type of PD, see Chapter 1) have reduced dopaminergic activity (^{18}F-dopa PET study in asymptomatic first-degree relatives of familial or isolated cases). Subtle parkinsonian clinical features, insufficient to fulfil Brain Bank criteria, were found in a subset of cases. Similar features occur in relatives of PARK6 patients.

◆ Relatives of PD patients who have a reduced sense of smell and/or abnormal transcranial ultrasound signals from the basal ganglia, show reduced dopamine activity on SPECT scanning.

◆ ^{18}F-dopa PET uptake is reduced in monozygotic twins (75% concordance) to a greater extent than in dizygotic twins (22% concordance), supporting a role for genetics in developing PD.

Postsynaptic dopamine imaging in parkinsonism

◆ Functional imaging of the postsynaptic dopamine system is possible using SPECT (ligands include IBZM, **55**) and PET (ligands include C11-raclopride).

◆ The postsynaptic neurones remain intact in idiopathic PD. Imaging of this area (e.g. ligands binding to the D2 receptor) therefore give a normal result (or a marginal increase from normal activity caused by upregulation in response to reduced presynaptic dopamine availability).

◆ Drugs which are antagonists at D2 receptors cause reduced uptake of the imaging ligand (i.e. the ligand has reduced binding to the receptor which is already occupied by the offending drug). This is the mechanism for most drugs which induce parkinsonism (e.g. neuroleptic agents).

◆ Parkinsonism occurs when D2 receptor occupancy by the drug is around 60–70%.

◆ Blockade by a drug at the D2 receptor may 'unmask' a very early case of idiopathic PD (see **33**).

◇ This occurs through blockade at a second neuronal site of dopaminergic transmission.

◇ Prolonged occupancy of D2 receptors, weeks or months after stopping the offending drug, has been shown.

◆ Abnormal D2 scans also occur in Parkinson-plus disorders.

◇ This occurs because the neuronal degeneration affects not only the presynaptic system (which is also affected in idiopathic PD, as described above) but also the postsynaptic system.

◇ In earlier stage Parkinson-plus disorders, the D2 SPECT results are often within the normal range or intermediate, preventing definitive radiological diagnosis.

◇ More correctly, the D2 SPECT results indicate the likelihood of a treatment response to dopaminergic therapy (at the time of the scan).

◇ Interpreting the postsynaptic scan assumes that dopamine-blocking drugs were not present at the time of the scan.

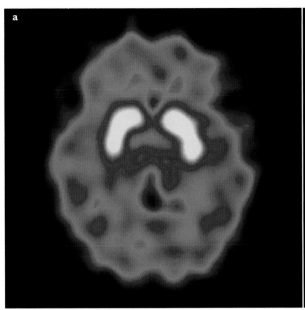 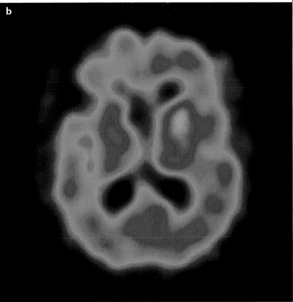

55 **Postsynaptic dopamine scanning.** Normal putamen and caudate activity is seen in the postsynaptic system in PD (a). This differs from presynaptic dopamine activity, which is abnormal in PD. Abnormal (reduced) activity is seen postsynaptically in conditions such as multiple system atrophy (b). However, these changes are more evident in later stage disease. In routine clinical practice, postsynaptic dopamine imaging does not reliably distinguish conditions such as MSA from PD.

◇ A positive (abnormal) scan is the most clear-cut result, while normal or intermediate results can occur in patients who later progress.
◆ Combining pre- and postsynaptic dopaminergic imaging to assist differential diagnosis has been undertaken with scans separated by 1 week (Beta-CIT and IBF) or conducted simultaneously (TRODAT and either IBZM or IBF).
◆ Antiparkinson medication should be omitted before postsynaptic dopamine imaging as follows:
◇ Short-term (overnight) stoppage of levodopa, selegiline, thrice daily DAs.
◇ Stop long-acting DAs (e.g. cabergoline) 36 hours pre-scan.
◇ Antidepressant therapy with selective serotonin reuptake inhibitors (SSRIs) should be stopped for 1 week.

Other types of functional neuroimaging in PD

◆ Serotonin binding (5-HT-1A) in the midbrain is reduced, which correlates with tremor severity (most patients were taking antiparkinson therapy at the time of their 11C-WAY PET study).
◆ Cholinergic activity is markedly reduced in frontal, temporal, and parietal cortex in patients with PD and dementia, compared to only very slight reductions from normal in patients with PD and no dementia (11C-MP4A PET study).

Functional neuroimaging in clinical drug trials

◆ Normal presynaptic scan results occur in a small proportion of patients entering clinical drug studies of antiparkinson therapy.
◇ 4% of 82 patients in a comparative trial of pramipexole and levodopa had normal Beta-CIT SPECT.
◇ 11% of 162 patients in a comparative trial of ropinirole and levodopa had normal ^{18}F-dopa PET.
◇ 14.7% of 142 patients in a trial comparing different doses of levodopa (against placebo) had normal Beta-CIT SPECT.
◇ Repeat functional neuroimaging remained normal (compared to further deterioration in patients with an initially abnormal scan result).

◇ Patients with normal scans had less therapy responsiveness in the levodopa study which contained a placebo group, but there was a therapy response in the normal scan patients in the studies without a placebo group.

◇ The results suggest alternative diagnoses (e.g. ET, dystonic tremor) or a variant of parkinsonism without presynaptic dopaminergic dysfunction.

◇ Increased congruence between baseline scan results and clinical diagnosis after follow-up to 4 years suggests that most of these cases had a nondegenerative disorder with features mimicking PD.

◆ Measurement of disease progression using functional neuroimaging has been used in several studies as a potentially more objective and more stable marker of disease severity than clinical scores.

◇ Sequential scanning showed a slower decline in ligand uptake in patients on DA therapy compared to patients on levodopa therapy (Beta-CIT SPECT and ^{18}F-dopa PET).

◇ Sequential scanning showed a slower decline in ligand uptake in patients on lower doses of levodopa compared to higher doses of levodopa (Beta-CIT SPECT).

◇ These studies suggest that longer-term DA therapy increases presynaptic dopamine turnover while the levodopa has a dose-dependent association with presynaptic dopamine turnover.

◇ There was no clinical correlate to suggest true neuroprotection.

Vascular parkinsonism and functional neuroimaging

◆ Normal (TRODAT) or near-normal (FP-CIT, Beta-CIT) or reduced (Beta-CIT) results are reported.

◇ Clinical criteria and case definitions vary amongst studies.

◇ Some studies excluded patients with structural imaging changes.

◇ Although group results distinguish between vascular parkinsonism and idiopathic PD, some individual cases with a clinical diagnosis of vascular parkinsonism have abnormal dopamine results.

◇ Coexistent vascular parkinsonism and idiopathic PD in individual cases may affect interpretation of functional neuroimaging results.

◆ Focal basal ganglia infarcts may cause 'punched out' areas which differ from the patterns of degenerative parkinsonism.

Clinical application of functional neuroimaging

◆ There is no overall consensus on the clinical utility of such imaging, but routine application of such imaging in all cases of PD is generally regarded as inappropriate.

◇ Cases of clearcut PD or clearcut ET do not require functional neuroimaging.

◇ Distinguishing PD from PSP or MSA is currently not feasible using presynaptic imaging, but postsynaptic imaging may be supportive.

◇ Recent brain bank studies suggest that clinical accuracy is high (90%) amongst patients thought to have idiopathic PD.

◇ Most misdiagnoses were for other forms of degenerative parkinsonism: MSA (6%), PSP (2%).

◇ Only 2% had postmortem diagnosis where presynaptic imaging would be expected to test normal.

◇ Diagnostic error rates from earlier in the clinical course are generally not available in brain bank studies of PD (which instead focus on last antemortem clinical diagnosis).

◆ There is no role for repeat functional neuroimaging to guide the patient on the progression rate of their disease.

◇ Test–retest variability is too high to allow such calculations in individual cases.

◆ Selected application in diagnostically difficult cases is supported by many specialists, based on:

◇ The finding of normal presynaptic scans in patients initially thought to have PD, in many clinical and research studies (and the fact that repeat scans at up to 4 years later are still normal).

◇ Later revision of clinical diagnosis in favour of baseline imaging results (reported in many clinical series).

◇ A high rate of change in clinical management has been attributed to presynaptic imaging results (but comparison to a control group has not been reported).

◇ The availability in Europe of FP-CIT (DaTSCAN, GE Healthcare) as a licensed product to aid differential diagnosis of PD from benign tremors.

Transcranial ultrasound

◆ Increased echogenicity is found from the substantia nigra region in PD.

◆ Combining this with other noninvasive tests (e.g. olfactory testing) can identify early disease and screen for preclinical disease.

Cardiac sympathetic nerve imaging

◆ Cardiac imaging determines the presence of cardiac sympathetic nerve dysfunction.

◆ Ligands include meta-iodobenzylguanidine (MIBG).

◆ The heart to mediastinum uptake ratio is calculated, and gives an index of cardiac sympathetic neurone loss.

◆ Results are abnormal (decreased) in PD, and correlate with dopamine transporter loss and (in some studies) with disease severity.

◆ Results are more likely to be normal in MSA and other degenerative parkinsonism, but testing is sensitive rather than specific.

Tremor recording

◆ Recording tremor frequency and amplitude may help distinguish PD tremor from other tremor types, including orthostatic tremor and psychogenic tremor.

◆ Techniques include electromyography and accelerometry (**56**).

56 **Tremor tracing in PD from accelerometry.** Tremor tracing from right wrist in a patient with PD for 20 years. The two channels represent different axes of movement (medial–lateral and superior–inferior) while the composite channel is an index of overall tremor severity. The tracing shows the typical reduction in tremor overnight (grey arrows), and fluctuating severity of tremor during the day (most severe around lunchtime; red arrow).

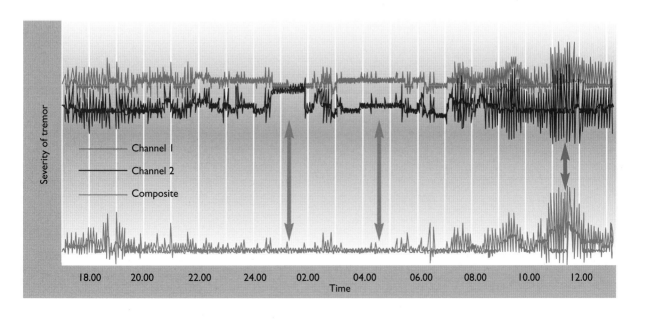

CHAPTER 4

Drug treatment of Parkinson's disease

Management principles

◆ Currently available drug treatments provide symptomatic benefit; none is proven as neuroprotective.

◆ Treatment is initiated when required from a functional viewpoint (this is variable between patients, and the decision requires patient and often carer input).

◆ Treatment is started at a variable point after the onset of symptoms (note symptom onset usually predates diagnosis).

◆ There are several initial treatment choices, each with advantages and disadvantages. The main choices are levodopa (with decarboxylase inhibitor), dopamine agonists (DAs), and monoamine oxidase B inhibitors (MAOB-Is). Anticholinergics and amantadine are sometimes used (but anticholinergics are generally better avoided as they may contribute to cognitive impairment, and can be difficult to withdraw because of rebound tremor). Drug choice is patient-specific depending on co-morbidities, biological age, and patient choice. Several randomized clinical trials compare drug classes, e.g. levodopa versus DAs, MAOB-Is versus placebo.

◆ PD is not a 'static' illness. Therefore, medications need to be titrated over time.

◆ In general, it is best to find the lowest dosage of any PD medication that will provide functional improvement.

◆ Not all motor symptoms of PD respond uniformly to pharmacological treatment. Bradykinesia and rigidity are most responsive to medications; postural instability is the least responsive to treatment; and pharmacological response to tremor is variable.

When to increase or add in therapy

◆ Signs of disease progression are increasing slowness, stiffness, and worsening tremor.

◆ Initial low-dose therapy with DA or levodopa is generally increased gradually for worsening symptoms and levels of function.

◆ Once initial therapy reaches the recommended maximum dose or maximally tolerated level, and addition of a second agent is required, a drug from a different class will become appropriate.

Signs of overtreatment

◆ Dopaminergic excess is characterized by confusion, hallucinations and involuntary movement (dyskinesia).

◆ Reduction of the dopaminergic therapy lowers such side-effects, but many patients prefer to tolerate mild visual hallucinations or dyskinesia as they find 'off' periods unpleasant and sometimes painful.

◆ Excessive sleep is common to all dopaminergic therapy and is dose related, and appropriate caution when driving or operating machinery is needed.

Note: *Most of the drug treatments described in this book are available internationally. Where a formulation is specific to either the USA or Europe, this is noted.*

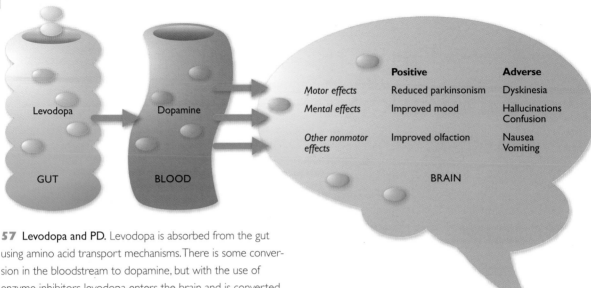

57 Levodopa and PD. Levodopa is absorbed from the gut using amino acid transport mechanisms. There is some conversion in the bloodstream to dopamine, but with the use of enzyme inhibitors levodopa enters the brain and is converted to dopamine for release from the presynaptic neurones. An overview of some effects of levodopa is shown.

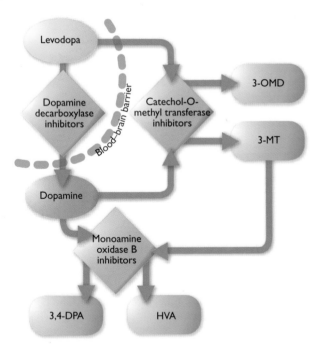

58 Levodopa metabolism and enzyme inhibitors.
The pathway for metabolism of levodopa to dopamine and its breakdown products (green) is shown: enzyme inhibitors (orange) function at three sites. Dopamine decarboxylase inhibitors work outside the blood–brain barrier and therefore promote the entry of levodopa to the brain for conversion to dopamine. The other enzyme inhibitors also supplement the effect of dopamine. The MAOB-Is function both on intrinsic dopamine and extrinsic levodopa. The COMT inhibitors function primarily as extenders to the duration of action of levodopa with much less effect on intrinsic dopamine.

Levodopa

- Levodopa (**57**) is a naturally occurring amino acid found in seedlings, pods, and broad (fava) beans.
- It was first introduced in the early 1970s and was a major therapeutic advance. Initially very high doses were given, and peripheral metabolism to dopamine caused intolerable nausea, dizziness, and postural hypotension, limiting its use.
- The discovery of peripheral decarboxylase inhibitors (carbidopa and benserazide) led to combined products of levodopa with decarboxylase inhibitors which dramatically alleviated adverse peripheral dopaminergic effects (**58**).
- Levodopa is currently the most effective treatment for parkinsonian symptom control and remains the 'gold standard'.
- Levodopa is available in many forms and formulations (**59**). Similar preparation names containing different amounts of active ingredients necessitate care by prescribers. At least 70 mg per day of the carbidopa is necessary to completely block peripheral decarboxylation (smaller doses have increased side-effects).
- The dosing is typically initiated at one 25/100 mg carbidopa/levodopa, referred to generically as co-careldopa, and by brand as Sinemet (or benserazide/levodopa, referred to generically as co-beneldopa, and by brand as Madopar) tablet three times daily and increased as necessary until clinical response is achieved.

Levodopa types, tablet strengths and uses

PREPARATION TYPE	TABLET STRENGTHS (mg)	CLINICAL APPLICATIONS
FAST OR 'IMMEDIATE' RELEASE Co-beneldopa dispersible e.g. Madopar dispersible (Europe)	12.5/50; 25/100	Taken in water; first morning dose; booster for sudden 'offs'
ORALLY DISINTEGRATING Co-careldopa eg. Parcopa (USA)	10/100; 25/100; 25/250	Standard management; dissolves without water
STANDARD RELEASE Co-careldopa eg. Sinemet (USA/Europe) and Co-beneldopa eg. Madopar (Europe)	12.5/50; 10/100; 25/100; 25/250	Standard management
CONTROLLED RELEASE Co-careldopa modified release eg. Sinemet CR (USA/Europe), and Co-beneldopa modified release eg. Madopar CR (Europe)	25/100; 50/200	Taken before bed to help overnight symptoms; alone or in combination with immediate-release levodopa for wearing off

59 Levodopa formulations. Levodopa is available in a range of dosages and tablet types.

- The dose of active levodopa is often used to calculate or refer to the total daily dose (e.g. 25/100 x 3 tablets per day = 300 mg levodopa).
- Smaller starting doses (e.g. 100 or 150 mg levodopa per day) are sometimes used in the UK (e.g. elderly patients with co-morbid illness, patients with psychiatric history), although this gives insufficient decarboxylase inhibitor.

- The recommended maximum dose of levodopa per day is 2000 mg.
- The main problems with levodopa result from a short half-life (90 minutes), which leads to peaks and troughs in serum (and therefore brain) levodopa levels (**60**) causing pulsatile rather than the more physiological continuous dopaminergic stimulation (**61**).

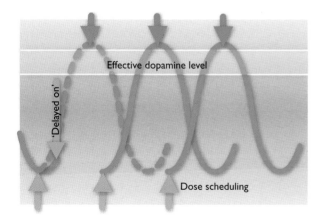

60 Fluctuations in levodopa levels. A dosing schedule results in peaks and troughs of serum and brain levodopa levels. The initial dose of levodopa in the morning may be associated with a 'delayed on' phenomenon (green arrow) until the medication begins to work. If the level exceeds the therapeutic window for an effective dopamine level, there may be associated involuntary movement referred to as peak dose dyskinesia (purple arrows).

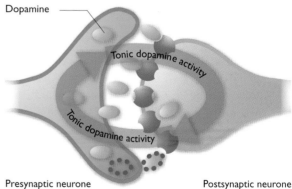

61 Normal dopamine flow. Dopamine is normally released constantly which creates a steady state between the pre- and postsynaptic neurones. This state is affected by PD where episodic delivery of medication results in changes at the postsynaptic receptor contributing to the development of motor fluctuations.

- The controlled-release (CR) preparations were developed to prolong the duration of action and provide smoother control and lessen the development of motor complications.
  - ◇ Sinemet CR is designed to release active ingredients over a 4–6-hr period via a slowly dissolving polymeric matrix and has approximately 70% bioavailability compared to standard (immediate) release. Dosage and dosing interval can be increased by up to 30%.
  - ◇ Madopar CR is transformed in the stomach to a mucoid body which delivers its content through a hydrated layer by diffusion.
- Lower bioavailability means that a 30% increase in dosing is sometimes recommended for CR preparations. In practice, patients are generally not guided to switch all their tablets from standard-release over to CR, or vice versa, as this is not helpful and the altered bioavailability will upset symptom control. In calculating the total dose per day, 100 mg of a CR preparation can be considered approximately equal to 70 mg.
- In clinical trials there was no difference in the development of motor fluctuations between immediate and CR preparations.
- The CR levodopa preparations may be subject to more variable gut absorption than immediate-release preparations, which can contribute to fluctuations in advanced disease.
- CR levodopa has a place as a nocturnal dose to help reduce overnight symptoms (DAs also have this role due to their longer half-life).
- Parcopa is an immediate-release, rapidly dissolving oral carbidopa/levodopa preparation available in the doses of immediate-release carbidopa/levodopa. It dissolves in the mouth without requiring water. However, its absorption is still intestinal and therefore the time to peak concentration is generally not faster than immediate-release carbidopa/levodopa.
- Occasionally, the immediate-release form is used to make a liquid preparation for PD patients with significant motor fluctuations by mixing 10 tablets of 25/100 mg carbidopa/levodopa with ½ teaspoon of ascorbic acid crystals and 1000 mL of distilled water. This preparation allows small and frequent dosing with the goal of relieving wearing-off symptoms without causing or worsening peak-dose dyskinesia.

- Abrupt discontinuation of levodopa should be avoided to prevent precipitation of a neuroleptic malignant-like syndrome characterized by rigidity, hyperthermia, altered consciousness, tachycardia, diaphoresis, and elevated creatine kinase.

Catechol-O-methyl transferase inhibitors

Entacapone

- Entacapone is a reversible, specific and mainly peripherally acting catechol-O-methyl transferase (COMT) inhibitor (see **58**).
- It decreases the metabolic loss of dopamine to 3 O-methyl dopa.
- It increases the half-life of levodopa by 30–50% so that the levodopa total daily dose may be reduced with no significant effect on the Cmax (peak concentration) or Tmax (time to Cmax).
- It is particularly indicated for patients experiencing end-of-dose 'wearing off', but can also be useful in patients with nonfluctuating disease.
- A single dose of 200 mg should be given together with each dose of levodopa up to ten times daily (up to eight times daily recommended in the USA).
- There is a small risk of developing diarrhoea after approximately 1 month of drug initiation, often requiring drug discontinuation. Entacapone should not be cut in half or chewed as it can discolour teeth yellow–orange. Warn patients also of benign orange discoloration of urine.

Stalevo

- A combination of entacapone, levodopa and carbidopa. It comes in four strengths containing 50, 100, 150 and 200 mg of levodopa.
- Using this combination product lowers the total number of pills required, which may aid therapy compliance.

Tolcapone

◆ Another predominantly peripherally acting COMT inhibitor, indicated for wearing off symptoms of PD.

◆ Available in two doses: 100 mg and 200 mg (USA only).

◆ It has a longer half-life than entacapone and is recommended to be taken no more than three times daily.

◆ May also cause diarrhoea generally after 1 month often requiring discontinuation of the drug. There have been three reported cases of acute liver failure potentially associated with tolcapone use. Therefore, frequent monitoring of liver function tests for 6 months and regularly thereafter is needed. This liver function monitoring is a requirement of the medicine regulators.

62 Dopamine agonists. Several oral and one subcutaneous agent are available, with different properties; apomorphine, for example, has the shortest half-life and cabergoline has the longest. Most involve hepatic metabolism.

Dopamine agonists

◆ Dopamine agonists (DAs) can be used as monotherapy in early disease or as an adjunct in later disease.

◆ DAs have a direct action on postsynaptic dopamine receptors.

◆ There are several different postsynaptic dopamine receptors (see **16**). D1, D2, and D3 are the principal subtypes. Further details of dopamine receptor types and affinities are described in Chapter 1. As DAs vary in their receptor affinity, switching between agents may be clinically advantageous.

◆ Several DAs are available with varying properties (summarized in **62**). However, the US Food and Drug Administration (FDA) has withdrawn pergolide because of its potential to cause fibrosis of the heart valves.

Drug treatment of Parkinson's disease

Pharmacokinetic properties of dopamine agonists

PREPARATION	ABSORPTION	TIME TO MAXIMUM PLASMA CONCENTRATION	BIOAVAILABILITY	ELIMINATION HALF-LIFE	CLEARANCE
Apomorphine (subcutaneous)	Very rapid	4–12 min	100%	33 mins	Extra-hepatic
Bromocriptine	Rapid	1–3 hr	6%	15 hr*	Hepatic
Cabergoline (Europe)	Rapid	0.5–4 hr	50–80%	63–68 hr#	Hepatic
Lisuride (Europe)	Rapid	0.2–1.2 hr	10–20%	1.3–2.5 hr	Hepatic
Pergolide (Europe)	55% absorbed	1–3 hr	20–60%	27 hr	Hepatic
Pramipexole	Rapid	1–3 hr	90%	8–12 hr+	Renal
Ropinirole	Rapid	1.5 hr	50%	6 hr	Hepatic

* Bromocriptine plasma elimination half-life is 3–4 hr for the parent drug and 50 hr for the inactive metabolites. The elimination of parent drug from plasma occurs biphasically, with a terminal half-life of about 15 hr.
\# In healthy volunteers.
\+ 8 hr in the young to 12 hr in the elderly.
Note: Pergolide is withdrawn in USA; pergolide and cabergoline second-line in Europe.

- When changing from one DA to another, overnight switching is usually effective if equivalent doses are used (**63**).
- Although less potent and subject to more side-effects than levodopa (see **13**), DAs have been proven in several trials to reduce and delay motor fluctuations, and delay the need to start levodopa. They are commonly used early as monotherapy, particularly in younger patients who are at higher risk of developing motor fluctuations.
- DAs can be broadly divided according to the presence of an ergot ring: ergot-based agonists (bromocriptine, pergolide, cabergoline, and lisuride) and non-ergot compounds (apomorphine, pramipexole, and ropinirole).
- *Adverse effects* occur as a class effect, the most common being nausea, dizziness, ankle swelling, confusion, hallucinations, and psychosis.
  - ◇ Adverse effects can be minimized by low initial doses and slow titration. Ropinirole has a starter pack which eases this process.
  - ◇ Idiosyncratic side-effects are reported more commonly with DAs then other PD medications and may include weight gain, compulsive behaviour, hypersexuality, and compulsive gambling. They have also been associated with excessive or sudden-onset sleepiness.
- ◇ Domperidone 10–20 mg three times daily helps to lessen nausea, dizziness, and postural hypotension (Europe).
- ◇ *Ergot adverse effects* (**64**) include pulmonary, pericardial, and retroperitoneal fibrosis and are reported for the ergot-based agonists. However, the site of action may be the 5-hydroxytryptamine 2B (5-HT2B) serotonin receptor rather than simply the presence of an ergot ring, as the ergot-derived DA lisuride does not cause fibrotic reactions and has a very low affinity for this receptor (**65**).
- ◇ Fibrotic heart valve changes detected on echocardiography (particularly the tricuspid valve) are reported in patients treated with pergolide and cabergoline. Monitoring of symptoms (in particular breathlessness), blood tests (erythrocyte sedimentation rate (ESR) and creatinine), chest X-ray, pulmonary function tests, and echocardiogram are recommended for patients taking these preparations long term. Pergolide has been withdrawn in the USA, and cabergoline and other ergot-derived DAs are considered second-line agents because of the issues over fibrotic complications.
- The transdermal agent rotigotine and CR ropinirole prolonged release are newer options. Both may reduce fluctuations by long duration of action.

63 Dopamine agonist conversion chart.

Dopamine agonists: approximate dose equivalents

BROMOCRIPTINE	CABERGOLINE	PERGOLIDE	PRAMIPEXOLE		ROPINIROLE
			SALT	BASE	
1 mg tid	0.5 mg od	0.125 mg tid	0.125 mg tid	0.088 mg tid	Starter pack then 1 mg tid
2.5 mg tid	1 mg od	0.25 mg tid	0.25 mg tid	0.18 mg tid	1 mg tid
5 mg tid	2 mg od	0.5 mg tid	0.5 mg tid	0.36 mg tid	2 mg tid
7.5 mg tid	3 mg od*	0.75 mg tid	0.75 mg tid	0.54 mg tid	3 mg tid
10 mg tid	4 mg od	1 mg tid	1 mg tid	0.7 mg tid	4 mg tid
12.5 mg tid	5 mg od	1.25mg tid	1.25mg tid	0.88 mg tid	6mg tid
15 mg tid	6 mg od	1.5 mg tid	1.5 mg tid	1.05 mg tid**	8mg tid

*Cabergoline maximum dose is now 3mg per day
**or 1.06mg if using 0.7 mg tablet + 2 × 0.18 mg tablets
Note: Pergolide is withdrawn in the USA; pergolide and cabergoline second-line in Europe.

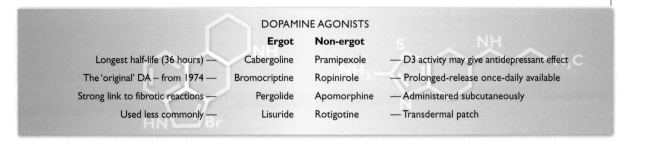

DOPAMINE AGONISTS		
	Ergot	**Non-ergot**
Longest half-life (36 hours) —	Cabergoline	Pramipexole — D3 activity may give antidepressant effect
The 'original' DA – from 1974 —	Bromocriptine	Ropinirole — Prolonged-release once-daily available
Strong link to fibrotic reactions —	Pergolide	Apomorphine — Administered subcutaneously
Used less commonly —	Lisuride	Rotigotine — Transdermal patch

64 **Dopamine agonists: ergot and non-ergot.** The broad division of DAs into ergot and non-ergot drugs and some key clinical features are shown.

65 **The 5-HT2B receptor and fibrotic complications.** Activity of several ergot-based DAs at the 5-HT2B serotonin receptor is considered important in the development of cardiac valve abnormalities and other fibrotic complications. Although lisuride is an ergot-derived DA, it does not have agonist activity at the 5-HT2B receptor and this is likely to be the reason that it has not been associated with such complications.

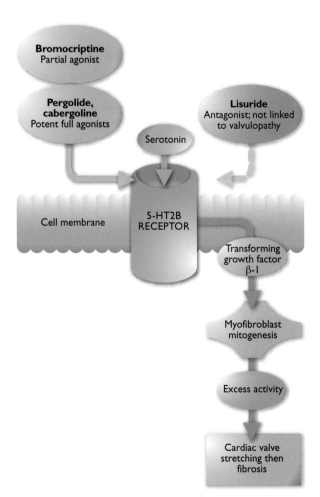

◆ *Apomorphine* is a DA which undergoes extensive first-pass metabolism and has to be administered parenterally. It can be given as a continuous waking day subcutaneous infusion (available in this form in Europe) or by bolus subcutaneous injections as needed as a 'rescue' therapy for wearing off. Currently, it is reserved for patients with advanced disease and significant motor fluctuations. The continuous delivery system smooths out off periods and dyskinesias, but may take a few weeks to reach a new 'steady state'. Oral DAs can usually be discontinued (sometimes a pre-bedtime single oral dose is given, as the infusion is usually discontinued overnight). A few patients have moved on to 24-hr infusions, and tolerance is not problematic. Oral drugs can often be reduced (gradually) and some patients successfully convert to apomorphine monotherapy in the daytime (but with overnight levodopa).

◆ For intermittent injections, efficacy is often felt within 10–20 minutes but lasts usually only for 1–1.5 hr. An extended outpatient/day case titration visit is often required to determine the optimal tolerated dose (see Chapter 8). Premedication with domperidone (available in Europe) for 3 days or trimethobenzamide 3–7 days prior to initiation is required to minimize GI side-effects.

◆ *Rotigotine* is a non-ergot D3/D2/D1 DA delivered transdermally over a 24-hr period.
  ◇ It is approved for the symptomatic treatment of early idiopathic PD (Europe and USA) and as an adjunct in later disease (Europe only).
  ◇ It is supplied as 2, 4, and 8 mg patches. The recommended starting dose is 2 mg/24 hr. This may be increased by 2 mg/24 hr every week until therapeutic response in achieved. The recommended top dose is 16 mg/24 hr.
  ◇ Aside from skin reactions, its side-effects are similar to those of other DAs: nausea, somnolence, and lower extremity oedema.

Monoamine oxidase inhibitors

- MAOB-Is prevent the breakdown of dopamine in the brain and inhibit the re-uptake of dopamine at the presynaptic receptor (see **58**).
- Enzyme inhibition is irreversible and therefore activity resumes only after new enzyme has been formed.
- They can be used as an early monotherapy and can prolong the time before levodopa is needed by approximately 9 months.
- In later disease adjunctive MAOB-I therapy can alleviate dose-related fluctuations and end-of-dose deterioration.

Selegiline
- Selegiline is well established, while rasagiline is a newer agent in the same class.
- Selegiline also comes in an oral lyophilisate formulation which dissolves completely within 10 s of being placed on the tongue. This is particularly indicated for patients with swallowing difficulties.
- The initial interpretation of selegiline studies was of some neuroprotection, but this failed to take account of symptomatic benefits.
- Selegiline became less popular after the United Kingdom Parkinson's Disease Research Group (UK-PDRG) study reported increased mortality, but other studies and meta-analysis found no increase in mortality with this drug class.
- Selegiline is relatively inexpensive.

Zydis selegiline (Zelapar)
- Zydis selegiline is a once-daily rapidly dissolving, under-the-tongue freeze-dried tablet formulation of selegiline approved as adjunct therapy for PD (USA) and as monotherapy or adjunct in Europe.
- It dissolves on contact with saliva, eliminating the need for water to aid in swallowing, which can be particularly useful in PD patients who often suffer from dysphagia.
- As a buccal administration, the tablet undergoes pregastric absorption, minimizing first-pass metabolism and producing high plasma concentrations of selegiline, with a three- to ten-fold reduction in amphetamine metabolites.

- A randomized, placebo-controlled, multicentre, double-blind, 12-week clinical trial evaluated the safety and efficacy of Zydis selegiline 15 (1.25 mg, titrated to 2.5 mg daily) as adjunctive therapy in PD patients who were experiencing motor fluctuations, and showed a significant reduction in percentage of off time among patients treated with Zydis selegiline. The total number of off hours was reduced by 2.2 hr/day in Zydis selegiline-treated patients compared with 0.6 hr/day in placebo-treated patients.
- It has not been evaluated in head-to-head studies with other adjunct PD therapies or as monotherapy in PD.

Rasagiline
- Rasagiline is a selective, second-generation, irreversible MAOB-I, with at least five times the potency of selegiline *in vitro* and in animal models.
- Rasagiline has demonstrated efficacy in one large, randomized double-blind, placebo-controlled trial as initial monotherapy in patients with early PD, and in two large, controlled trials as adjunctive treatment in levodopa-treated PD patients with motor fluctuations.
- Unlike selegiline, rasagiline is an aminoindan derivative with no amphetamine metabolites. A study comparing immediate with delayed therapy suggests that starting treatment early may be beneficial (**66**).
- The recommended dose is 1 mg per day. Rasagiline is available in Europe as 1 mg only, but in the USA as 0.5 mg and 1 mg, and is to be taken once per day.

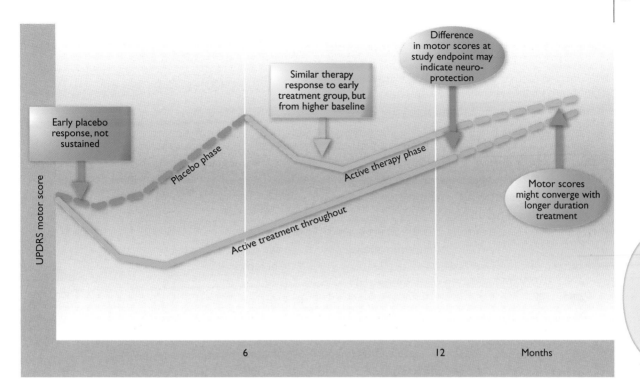

66 Delayed start in PD clinical trials. This type of trial design has been tested recently in the search for neuroprotective effect. Patients are randomized initially to active treatment or placebo, and subsequently all patients receive active therapy. A difference at the study end-point may suggest neuro-protection from earlier treatment start, particularly if motor scores remain divergent with longer duration of treatment.

Anticholinergics

◆ The use of anticholinergics in PD has declined in recent years due to adverse effects on cognition and the introduction of better alternative dopamine-sparing agents.

◆ Structurally related to atropine, these drugs block muscarinic receptors in the striatum, and inhibit the presynaptic carrier-mediated dopamine transport mechanism.

◆ Anticholinergics reduce tremor and rigidity, but have little effect on bradykinesia.

◆ They may be useful in reducing sialorrhoea.

◆ They can be used in drug-induced parkinsonism (e.g. in patients taking antipsychotic medication) if the offending drug cannot be withdrawn.

Amantadine

◆ Amantadine is a glutamate antagonist, originally developed as an antiviral agent.

◆ It enhances dopaminergic transmission and has mild antimuscarinic activity.

◆ It has modest antiparkinson effects with a mild improvement in bradykinesia, tremor, and rigidity.

◆ Its main use is in more advanced disease, as an antidyskinesia agent.

◆ Adverse effects include confusion, hallucinations, nervousness, poor concentration, peripheral oedema, and livedo reticularis.

◆ Usually amantadine is started at 100 mg twice per day with a top recommended dose of 200 mg twice per day.

Continuous dopaminergic stimulation

◆ Natural dopamine is released constantly without significant day–night (diurnal) variations.

◆ Dopamine replacement therapy should ideally replicate this, but the short duration of levodopa when given orally does not fulfil this need.

◆ Oral DAs have a longer duration of action, and help to smooth out the motor fluctuations inherent to levodopa therapy.

◆ Longer-acting oral DAs (e.g. ropinirole prolonged release) allow once-daily dosing, while transdermal, subcutaneous, and enteral routes (levodopa as Duodopa) offer more constant delivery (**67**, **68**).

◆ Allowing a small drop in overnight levels may prevent the development of tolerance (i.e. increasing doses required for the same effect) but the clinical significance of this is not certain.

◆ The way the patient times their medication influences plasma (and brain) levels and may contribute to motor fluctuations.

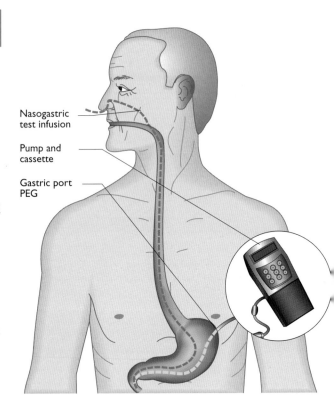

Nasogastric test infusion

Pump and cassette

Gastric port PEG

67 24-hour profile of antiparkinson therapy. Steady delivery of antiparkinson therapy fulfils the requirements of the continuous dopamine stimulation hypothesis. Avoiding fluctuating drug levels by infusions such as apomorphine and Duodopa, can help reduce motor fluctuations in late-stage disease. Longer-acting oral agents or transdermal delivery may prove helpful in a similar way. However, there remains a need for a long-acting agent with the efficacy of levodopa.

68 Duodopa infusion. An intestinal infusion of levodopa in the form of Duodopa as a concentrated gel, requires insertion of a percutaneous gastrostomy tube (yellow line) with the tip placed at the junction of the duodenum and jejunum. Treatment is typically given during the waking day, and this smooths out the fluctuations inherent in oral therapy in advanced disease.

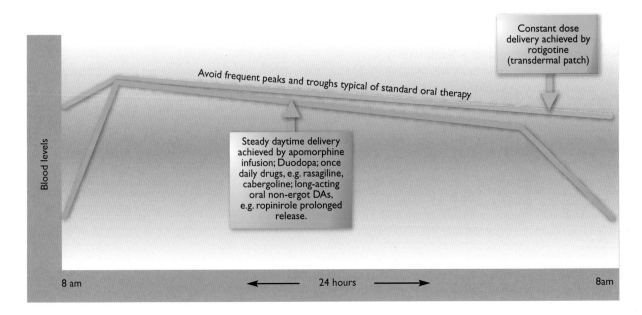

Constant dose delivery achieved by rotigotine (transdermal patch)

Avoid frequent peaks and troughs typical of standard oral therapy

Steady daytime delivery achieved by apomorphine infusion; Duodopa; once daily drugs, e.g. rasagiline, cabergoline; long-acting oral non-ergot DAs, e.g. ropinirole prolonged release.

Blood levels

8 am   ⟵ 24 hours ⟶   8am

CHAPTER 5

Nonmotor features of Parkinson's disease

Cognitive impairment

The latest Diagnostic and Statistical Manual of Mental Disorders (DSM) defines dementia as, 'The development of multiple cognitive deficits that include memory impairment and at least one of the following cognitive disturbances: aphasia, apraxia, agnosia, or disturbance in executive functioning. The cognitive deficits must be sufficiently severe to cause impairment in occupational or social functioning and must represent a decline from a previously higher level of functioning.'

◆ Dementia is thus largely a clinical diagnosis corroborated by psychometric testing.

◆ The four cognitive domains (**69**) that can be affected include:

◇ *Recent memory* – the ability to learn, retain, and retrieve newly acquired information.

◇ *Language* – the ability to comprehend and express verbal information.

◇ *Visual spatial function* – the ability to manipulate and synthesize nonverbal, geographic, or graphic information.

◇ *Executive function* – the ability to perform abstract reasoning, solve problems, plan for future events, mentally manipulate more than one idea at a time, maintain mental focus in the face of distraction, or shift mental effort easily.

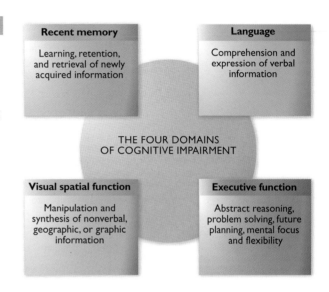

69 Cognitive impairment. The four domains of cognitive impairment which are relevant to PD are shown.

Incidence and prevalence of dementia in PD

◆ The definition and frequency of dementia in PD are controversial.

◆ Incidence rates for PD dementia range from 4.2–9.5% per year. Depending on the sample population and criteria used, the prevalence rate of PD dementia ranges from 10–40%.

◆ In a population-based study of PD with and without dementia, the crude PD prevalence was 99.4/100,000 and the crude PD dementia prevalence was 41.1/100,000.

◆ The prevalence of dementia increased with age, from 0 (for <50 years of age) to 787.1/100,000 (for >79 years of age). Interestingly, the major difference between PD patients with and without dementia was a later age of onset of motor manifestations in PD with dementia.

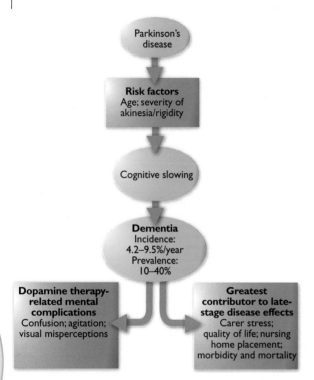

70 Risks and consequences of dementia. With advancing disease dementia is more common and becomes a significant contributor to the management difficulties of many patients.

◆ There is reasonable consensus that the overall risk of developing global cognitive impairment in PD increases with age and the severity of akinesia/rigidity (**70**).

◆ The following have not consistently been shown to be risk factors: age of onset of motor symptoms; longer duration of illness; gender; low level of formal education; depressive symptoms; psychosis precipitated by levodopa; and a family history of dementia.

◆ By the year 2050, it is projected that the number of individuals over 65 will increase to 1.1 billion worldwide. As a consequence, the number of dementia cases may reach 37 million. By 2050, the total cost of dementia as an illness is estimated to reach $383 billion in the USA.

◆ In PD, dementia may be the single most important factor limiting the application of standard pharmacotherapy for bradykinesia, rigidity, and tremor.

◆ PD patients with concomitant dementia are particularly prone to the development of dopamine-induced confusion, agitation, and visual misperceptions.

◆ The sequelae of dementia are now the most important contributors in late-stage PD to carer stress, poor quality of life, early nursing home placement, morbidity, and mortality.

Neurobiology of dementia in PD

◆ The pathology of PD affects function primarily in the striatum (caudate and putamen) and secondarily in the frontal cortex (**71**).

◆ Cell loss in the following areas contributes to cognitive decline in PD: the substantia nigra pars compacta; nucleus basalis of Meynert; locus coeruleus; and limbic cortex.

◇ Reliable correlations have been demonstrated between clinical (motor) stage and dopamine metabolism in the putamen but not the caudate nucleus. Conversely, metabolism in the caudate, but not the putamen, correlates with impairment in a cognitive task (delayed verbal recall). This so-called functional division of the striatum is, perhaps, the main reason for the relative predominance of motor over cognitive symptoms due to loss of dopamine in uncomplicated PD.

◇ However, cholinergic networks mediate aspects of memory and attention in animal and human studies, and are at least as damaged in PD patients as in patients with Alzheimer's disease. In autopsy series, striking cell loss is found in the nucleus basalis of Meynert. Nicotinic cholinergic receptor binding in the putamen is also decreased in PD.

◇ The noradrenergic system is said to play a major role in aspects of attentional control and depressed mood, both of which influence cognition, as well as the late-stage gait difficulties of PD related to postural instability, frequent falls, and freezing.

◇ Finally, cell loss from the raphe nuclei leads to deficiency in the almost ubiquitous serotonin projection systems that help regulate mood. Some form of depression is experienced by at least 40% of patients with PD at some point in their clinical course. Mood fluctuators and patients with clinically apparent mood changes during their motor 'on' and 'off' states may be more likely to have dementia.

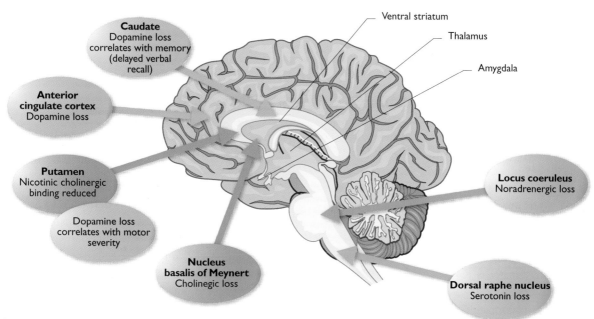

Caudate
Dopamine loss
correlates with memory
(delayed verbal
recall)

Ventral striatum

Thalamus

Amygdala

Anterior
cingulate cortex
Dopamine loss

Putamen
Nicotinic cholinergic
binding reduced

Locus coeruleus
Noradrenergic loss

Dopamine loss
correlates with motor
severity

Nucleus
basalis of Meynert
Cholinegic loss

Dorsal raphe nucleus
Serotonin loss

71 Neurobiology of dementia in PD. Damage to neurological pathways involving more than one neurotransmitter is considered important. There is involvement of the dopamine, acetylcholine, serotonin, and noradrenergic systems. A contribution from the serotonin system associated with depression can influence the presentation of dementia features.

Chemical neurotransmitters affected in PD

☐ Dopamine
☐ Acetylcholine
☐ Serotonin
☐ Noradrenaline

Cognitive dysfunction in PD

◆ Disturbances of frontal executive function remain consistently among the earliest cognitive manifestations of PD.

◆ Patients (and more often their carers) often report that they are having problems with decision making, planning, and completion of goal-directed behaviours.

◆ For individuals in whom cognition is less affected early on, with a good motor response to levodopa, cognitive changes may proceed in at least three ways: they may continue to remain relatively unscathed throughout their clinical course with isolated or small groups of deficits; they may begin to develop increasing behavioural, mood, and cognitive difficulties with a predominance of frontal lobe dysfunction; or they may develop more severe and global cognitive deficits.

◆ If early in the clinical course of parkinsonism, cognitive difficulties are already noted, concomitant Alzheimer's disease with PD, or one of the Parkinson-plus syndromes (fronto-temporal dementia with parkinsonism, PSP) or DLB should be considered.

General treatment

◆ General approaches to treating the consequences of established dementia in PD follow the same principles applied to other geriatric populations and other dementing illnesses.

◆ Infections, metabolic, and endocrine derangements, hypoperfusion states, and social stress are also common precipitating factors for worsened mental status and should be addressed or recognized.

◆ Substance abuse, including reliance on over-the-counter preparations containing antihistamines, may be under-appreciated, especially in individuals who are living alone.

◆ Medications with central nervous system (CNS) effects such as narcotics, sedative hypnotics, antidepressants, anxiolytics, and antihistamines should be avoided, or used sparingly.

◆ Many other commonly prescribed medications, including antiemetics, antispasmodics for the bladder, H2 receptor antagonists, antiarrhythmic agents, antihypertensive agents, and nonsteroidal anti-inflammatory agents, may also cause cognitive impairment.

Specific treatments

◆ Cholinesterase inhibitors.

◇ Four members of this class of compounds are currently FDA approved for the treatment of mild to moderate Alzheimer's disease. Tacrine does not have Europe-wide approval. Rivastigmine is now also licensed (in the USA and Europe) for treatment of dementia associated with PD.

◇ Tacrine, donepezil, rivastigmine, and galantamine are all inhibitors of the enzyme acetylcholinesterase (AChE) and, in theory, help repair brain cholinergic deficits by increasing the amount of acetylcholine available for binding in the synaptic cleft to cholinergic receptors.

◇ The pharmacokinetic properties and *in vivo* ability to modulate cholinergic networks of each of these compounds are quite different (**72**).

72 Cholinesterase inhibitors. There are four drugs in this class currently approved by the FDA.

◇ Each of these compounds has shown comparable efficacy in maintaining Alzheimer's Disease Assessment Scale-cognitive portion (ADAS-cog) scores above baseline in double-blind controlled studies in Alzheimer's disease.

◇ Brain metabolism has been shown by FDG-PET to increase in tandem with clinical benefit.

◇ In observational studies, long-term use of cholinesterase inhibitors translated into a 2-year delay in admission to nursing homes.

◇ For all the cholinesterase inhibitors, the most common side-effects are GI distress (nausea, diarrhoea, vomiting), fatigue, insomnia, and muscle cramps.

◇ Theoretical concerns about worsening seizures, asthma, conduction abnormalities, chronic obstructive pulmonary disease, and peptic ulcer disease, seem not to have materialized as significant adverse events despite the thousands of individuals with Alzheimer's disease who have now been exposed to these drugs.

Cholinesterase inhibitors

	Tacrine	Donepezil	Rivastigmine	Galantamine
CHOLINESTERASE INHIBITION	Noncompetitive reversible	Noncompetitive reversible	Noncompetitive reversible; most potent	Competitive reversible; least potent
BUTYRYL CHOLINESTERASE	+	Negligible	+	Negligible
NICOTINIC ACETYLCHOLINE RECEPTOR INHIBITION	–	–	–	Allosteric modulation
METABOLISM	Hepatic CYP450	Hepatic CYP450	Renal	Hepatic renal
PLASMA HALF-LIFE	2–4 hr	~70 hr	~1 hr; enzyme dissociation time 8 hr	~6 hr
DOSING	qid	od	bid	bid
INITIAL DOSE	5 mg	2.5 mg	1.5 mg	4 mg
MAXIMUM DOSE	160 mg	10 mg	12 mg	32 mg
WARNING LABEL	Hepatotoxicity	–	–	–
DRUG INTERACTIONS	+	+	None known	+

◇ Recently, investigators have begun to consider the potential of these compounds for treating dementia in PD. This change was encouraged by slow confirmation of the more benign side-effect profiles of the last three cholinesterase inhibitors, and reports of better efficacy in treating the cognitive and neuropsychiatric concomitants of DLB.

◇ The first randomized, double blind, placebo-controlled, crossover study reported that 14 PD subjects with cognitive impairment showed improvement in the Mini Mental State Examination (MMSE) and the Clinician's Interview Based Impression of Change (CIBIC) with donepezil compared to placebo. Motor UPDRS subscores did not worsen during donepezil treatment. Three patients had improved scores on delusions, two on hallucinations, one on agitation, six on depression, and five on apathy.

◇ Another randomized, double-blind, placebo-controlled, crossover study in 22 subjects with PD and dementia receiving either donepezil followed by identical placebo or vice versa showed donepezil was well tolerated. There was no worsening of PD symptoms as measured by the motor sections of the UPDRS. There may be a modest benefit on aspects of cognitive function. The possible clinical benefit was reflected in only one of the cognitive scales used in this study.

◇ Recently, 541 PD patients with dementia were enrolled in a double-blind study comparing rivastigmine versus placebo. The rivastigmine-treated patients had a mean improvement of 2.1 points in the ADAS-cog compared to a 0.7 point worsening in the placebo group.

◇ A single trial using nicotinic patches did not show any benefit in either Alzheimer's disease or PD.

◇ Other possible approaches to improving cholinergic function in the brain, such as dietary supplementation with cholinergic precursors (lecithin) and administration of cholinergic receptor agonists (bethanechol, milameline, tasaclidine), have not been found to be useful in Alzheimer's disease, and at this point are unlikely to be tried in patients with PD dementia.

◆ Other strategies.

◇ Recently, memantine, a noncompetitive antagonist of the NMDA receptor, was approved in the USA as therapy for the treatment of moderate to severe Alzheimer's disease. The drug was well tolerated by patients with cognitive decline and improved the cognitive status and day-to-day function of Alzheimer patients. While there have been some reports showing memantine improves motor symptoms of PD, it has not yet been reported to improve PD dementia in a double-blind, placebo-controlled trial.

◇ Attempts to compensate for noradrenergic deficits in PD have been reported. The first study trialled L-threo-3,4-dihydroxyphenyl-serine (L-DOPS) in individuals with late-stage PD. A moderate improvement in gait freezing, bradyphrenia, and depression was observed; the benefit has not been repro-duced. The second trial consisted of nine PD patients treated with naphtoxazine (SDZ-NVI-085), a selective noradrenergic alpha-1 agonist. This seemed to improve subject per-formance on two classic tests of frontal lobe function: the Stroop and Odd-Man-Out tests.

◇ Oestrogen replacement therapy (ERT) may be a reasonable protective strategy for the development of dementia in women who have PD. The effect of ERT on the risk of development of dementia was investigated in 87 women with PD without dementia, 80 women with PD with dementia, and 989 healthy women without dementia. ERT did not affect the risk of PD, but appeared to be protective for the development of dementia arising within the setting of PD (OR 0.22; 95% CI, 0.05–1.0). Another large survey of all PD nursing home residents in five US states, comparing women residents on ERT versus those who were not, found PD residents on oestrogen to be less cognitively impaired.

◇ There are no data at present on the ability of purported enhancers of mitochondrial function, such as coenzyme Q10 (CoQ10) or creatine, to improve cognitive function in PD.

◇ Based on epidemiological studies showing lower prevalence or delayed onset of dementia, anti-inflammatory agents may be beneficial in the treatment of dementia.

Nonmotor features of Parkinson's disease

Psychiatric complications

- Psychotic symptoms are common in patients suffering from PD.
- Visual hallucinations (**73**) are the most common manifestation, occurring in approximately 30% of patients with PD.
- The hallucinations are usually comprised of complex forms: they often appear to move, and occur almost exclusively when the eyes are open.
- Auditory (10%) and tactile (8%) hallucinations may also occur with PD, but usually exist in concert with visual hallucinations.
- Although PD patients with hallucinations typically have intact reality testing (benign hallucinosis), at least 5% experience delusions and hallucinations unaccompanied by insight.
- Unlike delirium, PD-related hallucinations occur in the setting of a clear sensorium.
- Socioeconomic sequelae of PD-related psychosis include higher caregiver stress, increased rates of nursing home placement, and dramatically worsened prognosis in extended care facilities.

- Unfortunately, hallucinations in PD tend to persist and, not uncommonly, may worsen over time.
- Multiple risk factors for PD-related hallucinations have been identified.
  - ◇ Psychotic symptoms usually occur in cases of advanced, chronically treated PD.
  - ◇ All anti-PD medications have been implicated in the development of hallucinations. Chronic exposure to multiple anti-PD medications appears to be a particularly potent risk factor for their occurrence.
  - ◇ Low MMSE scores, and high UPDRS scores (see chapter 6) are also associated with the presence of hallucinations.
  - ◇ Vivid dreams and nightmares, which in some studies have been correlated with duration of levodopa therapy, may also be harbingers of PD-related hallucinations.

Pathophysiology

- Excessive dopaminergic activity, probably in mesocortical and mesolimbic systems, appears to play a role in the generation of hallucinations.
- There are experimental suggestions that chronic stimulation may cause persistent sensitization of dopamine receptors, thereby causing susceptibility to psychotic phenomena.
- Exogenous dopamine is clearly not the only factor in the pathophysiology of hallucinations.
- The relationship between serotonergic systems and PD-related psychosis remains unclear. The purported efficacy of atypical antipsychotic agents, such as clozapine and quetiapine, without worsening motor function, have been partly attributed to their affinity for 5-HT receptors.
- Some neuropathological specimens of patients with DLB indicate that levels of choline acetyltransferase (ChAT) were lower, and the ratio of 5-hydroxyindoleacetic acid to ChAT was higher, in hallucinating patients than in non-hallucinating patients. Marked degeneration of cholinergic neurones is evident in the brains of PD patients, possibly to a greater degree than that seen in patients with AD.
- The relationship between sleep disturbances and hallucinations is another fertile area of study. Vivid dreams preceded or accompanied 61.3% of the hallucinations experienced by PD patients in one study.

```
        Hallucinations
        in Parkinson's
           disease

      Risk factors
   Chronic exposure to
   multiple antiparkinson
   medications; low MMSE
   scores; high parkinson
   motor scores; vivid
   dreams

VISUAL 30%    AUDITORY 10%    TACTILE 8%
Complex and   Usually occur in conjunction with
moving; often people    visual hallucinations
or animals; occur
with eyes open

      Pathophysiology
   Excess dopaminergic
   activity; possible links to
   serotonin and cholinergic
   systems; low levels of
   choline acetyltransferase;
   dysfunction of visual
   networks: processing and
   categorization
```

73 Hallucinations in PD. These are typically visual but other types are described. Insight is retained in 95% of occurrences.

- Visual dopaminergic systems, even at the level of the retina, are impaired in PD patients, but no definite functional correlate of this pathology has been identified.
- The multiple neurochemical and neuropsychological abnormalities that are associated with psychosis in PD suggest that no single brain structure accounts for the PD-related hallucinations.

General treatment

- As in any geriatric and/or neurological patient, urinary and pulmonary infections, metabolic and endocrine derangements, cerebral hypoperfusion states and even social stressors such as changes in the environment are potential precipitating factors for delirium and psychosis in PD. A search for these correctable causes is always required.
- Another easily ignored aetiology is the addition of medications with CNS effects such as narcotics, hypnotics, antidepressants, anxiolytics and any pharmacological agent that crosses the blood–brain barrier, including anti-PD medications.
- If psychotic symptoms persist despite the withdrawal of psychotropic medications, anti-PD medications are then gradually reduced or, if possible, discontinued.
- Most authorities slowly 'peel off' anti-PD drugs in the following order: anticholinergic agents, selegiline, amantadine, DAs, then COMT-Is, and finally, levodopa.
- Often, reliance on the regular/short-acting formulation of levodopa is preferred over the sustained-release formulation because its pharmacokinetics are more predictable and the shorter half-life means less potential for the cumulative side-effects of repeated dosing.
- If psychosis improves, the patient is then maintained on the lowest possible dose of anti-PD medication. However, withdrawal of anti-PD drugs usually worsens parkinsonism and may not be tolerated.

Atypical antipsychotic (AA) agents

- The choice of an AA agent is based largely on its ease of use and side-effect profile, as most antipsychotic agents, with few exceptions, have comparable efficacy in improving psychosis.

- The main difference in the antipsychotic agents lies in their propensity to worsen motor functioning in this frail and already vulnerable population.
- Thus far, six drugs have been marketed in the USA and Europe as 'atypical': clozapine, risperidone, olanzapine, quetiapine, ziprasidone, and aripiprazole.
- The use of an AA agent may allow the clinician to control psychosis with fewer motor side-effects and, in some cases, without the need for cutting back on anti-PD medications.
- It remains unclear whether antipsychotic medications should be continued once they are initiated. There are some data that show persistence of hallucinations in PD patients with drug-induced psychosis after its initial occurrence.
- One study prospectively followed PD patients on successful long-term treatment with quetiapine or clozapine as these drugs were withdrawn. The study was aborted after enrolment of only six patients due to an unacceptably high rate of psychosis recurrence (five patients, 83%). Psychosis recurred within 2 months of the end of each taper.
- Clozapine.
  ◇ The cumulative experience of all open-label reports on clozapine in parkinsonism involving over 400 patients has been surprisingly consistent. Low doses are required (average of 25 mg/day).
  ◇ A meta-analysis of all large clozapine reports on psychosis in PD showed an 85% improvement rate with acceptable tolerance. Most importantly, clozapine did not worsen motor symptoms. In some reports, it improved tremor.
  ◇ Clozapine remains difficult to use because of its potential for inducing agranulocytosis. The problem is idiosyncratic, so that even the small doses used in PD do not exempt patients from this side-effect.
  ◇ In the USA, for the first 6 months, each patient on clozapine undergoes a weekly white blood cell (WBC) count, verified by the pharmacy, and can receive only 1 week's supply of the drug at a time. After 6 months the process becomes bi-weekly. In the UK and Europe, similar strict monitoring is mandatory through case registration.

◆ Risperidone.
  ◇ Risperidone causes dose-related problems typical of conventional neuroleptics such as prolactin elevation and acute dystonic reactions.
  ◇ Almost all reports concerning risperidone in PD have involved open-label studies.
  ◇ Unfortunately, the studies showed mixed results. A meta-analysis of 82 PD patients treated with risperidone revealed that 23 (28%) experienced motor worsening.
◆ Olanzapine. This is a thiobenzodiazepine of similar chemical structure to clozapine. However, the 2002 Movement Disorders Society Task Force evidence-based review on the treatment of psychosis in PD concluded that there is 'insufficient evidence to demonstrate efficacy of olanzapine in drug-induced psychosis', and it carries an 'unacceptable risk of motor deterioration' even at 'low conventional doses', based on disappointing double-blind trial results in PD patients with hallucinations.
◆ Quetiapine.
  ◇ Quetiapine is a dibenzothiazepine with the closest pharmacological resemblance to clozapine but without the risk of agranulocytosis.
  ◇ Unfortunately, quetiapine has been subject to only one small, single-centre double-blind trial.
  ◇ However, several open-label reports involving over 200 PD patients give a fairly solid, positive impression of the drug's standing as an AA agent.
  ◇ Quetiapine appears to be slightly less effective than clozapine against psychosis. Unlike clozapine, it does not improve tremor, and may induce mild motor worsening. But, unlike olanzapine and risperidone, no reported motor worsening on quetiapine has precipitated hospitalization.
  ◇ The mean daily dose was generally below 75 mg/day.
◆ Ziprasidone.
  ◇ Ziprasidone has a higher affinity for 5-HT2 than D2 receptors. There has been no report of its use in the PD population.
  ◇ A panel of expert psychiatrists reviewing all available data on ziprasidone use in schizophrenia concluded that its extrapyramidal

syndrome profile is 'better than risperidone, the same as olanzapine but not quite as good as quetiapine or clozapine'.
◆ Aripiprazole.
  ◇ Aripiprazole is the only AA agent that is a partial agonist at the D2 and 5-HT1A receptors and an antagonist at 5-HT2A receptors. It also has a high 5-HT2/D2 ratio and may therefore carry a low risk of extrapyramidal side-effects while alleviating psychosis in PD-vulnerable populations.
  ◇ The preliminary experience, however, is mixed but not very encouraging. In one report, only two out of eight PD patients experienced near-complete resolution of their psychotic symptoms with aripiprazole. The other six patients discontinued aripiprazole within 40 days, two due to motor worsening.
  ◇ Controlled studies are currently under way to definitively evaluate the safety and tolerability of aripiprazole use in parkinsonian patients.

Other agents and treatments

◆ Ondansetron. In an open-label trial of 16 PD patients using ondansetron, a 5-HT3 receptor blocker, marked improvement in the areas of visual hallucinations, confusion, and functional impairment was found with no effect on UPDRS scores. These positive findings have not been universally reproduced.
◆ Acetylcholinesterase inhibitors.
  ◇ In an open-label study, five of seven PD patients with dementia had complete resolution of their hallucinations when treated with tacrine; the other patients showed improvement. None of the patients had worsening of their UPDRS motor scores.
  ◇ In addition to being an AChE inhibitor, galantamine also potentiates nicotinic acetylcholine neurotransmission. In an open-label trial in patients with PD and dementia, seven of the nine patients with hallucinations experienced amelioration of their hallucinations with galantamine.
  ◇ Rivastigmine is an AChE inhibitor that also inhibits the activity of butyryl cholinesterase. One open-label study of rivastigmine for PD-related psychosis and cognitive impairment

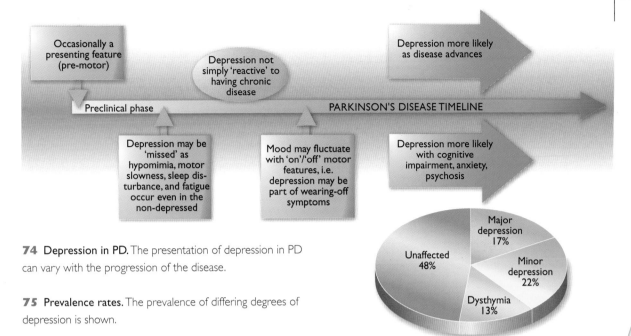

74 Depression in PD. The presentation of depression in PD can vary with the progression of the disease.

75 Prevalence rates. The prevalence of differing degrees of depression is shown.

involved 15 patients. In the 12 subjects who completed the study, hallucinations, sleep disturbance, and carer stress were improved. Motor scores did not worsen.

◇ Reports about successful treatment of psychosis in DLB using donepezil suggest that this agent might be helpful in PD. One study followed eight PD patients on 5 mg of donepezil per night, and reported significant improvement in psychotic symptoms in all patients. Another open study of donepezil observed three patients with visual hallucinations that improved with donepezil, but one patient experienced treatment-emergent delusions that disappeared when donepezil was discontinued.

◆ Electroconvulsive therapy (ECT). This is most commonly used for treatment-resistant psychiatric disorders. It has also been reported to improve motor symptoms of PD. In general, ECT's effects are short-lived, and repeated treatments and/or pharmacological augmentation are required to maintain any benefits. ECT has not been extensively studied in PD-related psychosis. There have been some scattered reports of success. It should probably be reserved for patients who are unresponsive to, or intolerant of, other treatments, especially if psychosis is associated with severe depression.

Behavioural dysfunction

Depression

◆ Depressive symptoms may occur at any stage of PD and are a major factor related to poor quality of life for both the patient and their carer (**74**).

◆ It may precede or occur along with or after the onset of motor symptoms.

◆ The prevalence rates of depressive disorders in Parkinson's disease vary widely and range from 2.7% to over 90%. In a meta-analysis of 36 articles, the weighted prevalence in PD was 17% for major depression, 22% for minor depression and 13% for dysthymia (**75**).

◆ Factors correlated consistently with depression include advanced disease, cognitive impairment, anxiety, and psychosis.

◆ Depressed PD patients may experience less guilt and self-blame but greater anxiety, cognitive deficits, irritability, and suicidal ideation without suicidal behaviour compared to depressed non-PD patients. Symptoms tend to worsen over time and amplify motor and other impairments.

◆ Changes in mood are associated with medication 'on' or 'off' states.

◆ Degeneration of mesolimbic dopamine, norepinephrine, and serotonergic pathways, along with degeneration of orbital-frontal circuits, locus coeruleus, dorsal raphe nuclei, and ventral tegmental area, are postulated to be associated with depression.

- There is hypometabolism in the caudate and orbital inferior frontal lobe in FDG-PET scans of depressed PD patients.
- Depression is probably not just a reaction to PD disability as depression is more common and more severe in PD compared to other chronic, disabling conditions such as rheumatoid arthritis or macular degeneration.
- PD depression may be underdiagnosed as some symptoms of depression are regular features of PD such as masked facies, psychomotor retardation, sleep disruption, fatigue.
- Depression scales which may be completed by PD patients include: Becks Depression Inventory, Geriatric Depression Scale, Zung Self-Rating Scale, Hospital Anxiety and Depression Scale, and the Center for Epidemiologic Studies Depression Scale. Clinician-completed rating scales such as the Hamilton Depression Rating Scale and the Montgomery-Ashberg Depression Scale are validated for use in the PD population.
- Work-up should include: complete blood count (CBC); liver function tests; serum testosterone levels (in men); thyroid function tests (symptoms of hypothyroidism include fatigue, irritability, motor retardation, decreased concentration); drug inventory (e.g. beta-blockers can cause depressive side-effects); identification of motor fluctuations (nonmotor symptoms can occur in the 'off' states).
- There are only a few randomized clinical trials assessing the efficacy and safety of antidepressants in PD.
  - ◇ Amitryptyline, desipramine, and nortriptyline all demonstrate antidepressive effects in PD.
  - ◇ In three randomized trials comparing tricyclic antidepressants (TCAs) and selective serotonin reuptake inhibitors (SSRIs) in depressed PD patients, amitriptyline was superior in one, and fluoxetine or sertraline was equally as efficacious as amitriptyline in the two other trials.
  - ◇ Mirtazapine, a selective norepineprhine reuptake inhibitor (SNRI) was superior to placebo in 20 depressed PD patients. Sedation was found to be inversely correlated with dosage. Mirtazapine may possibly improve tremor or dyskinesias.
  - ◇ Nefazodone was similar to fluoxetine in improving depression.

- SSRIs and TCAs may be the most useful drugs for the treatment of depression in PD, but SSRIs may be better tolerated (**76**).
- Amoxapine and lithium can cause or worsen parkinsonism and should be avoided.
- Nonselective MAOB-Is, such as isocarboxazid, phenelzine, and tranylcypromine, should also be avoided in levodopa-treated patients because of the risk of hypertensive crisis.
- Sedating TCAs (amitriptyline and doxepin) may be beneficial in PD patients with insomnia.
- Tertiary amine TCAs (amitriptyline, doxepin, and imipramine) may be beneficial in PD patients with concomitant bladder hyperactivity and drooling, but harmful in patients with confusion, hallucinations, hypotension, and excessive daytime sleepiness (EDS).
- Citalopram, escitalopram, fluoxetine, fluvoxamine, paroxetine, sertraline, nefazodone (SSRIs), bupropion (a DA reuptake inhibitor), venlafaxine (inhibits 5-HT and norepinephrine reuptake), have all been described in PD.
- ECT is effective in improving depressive symptoms and transiently improving motor symptoms as well.
- It remains unclear if repetitive transcranial magnetic stimulation also improves depressive and motor symptoms of PD.

Anxiety

- Anxiety disorders are classified into the following: panic disorder without agoraphobia; panic disorder with agoraphobia; agoraphobia without panic disorder; specific phobia; social phobia; obsessive–compulsive disorder (OCD); post-traumatic stress disorder; acute stress disorder; generalized anxiety disorder (GAD); anxiety disorder due to a general medical condition; substance-induced anxiety disorder; and anxiety disorder not otherwise specified.
  - ◇ A *panic attack* is a discrete period of a sudden onset of intense apprehension, fearfulness, or terror, often associated with feelings of impending doom. During these attacks, symptoms such as shortness of breath, palpitations, chest pain, choking or smothering sensations, and fear of 'going crazy' or losing control are present. In *panic disorder*, there is a persistent concern over recurrent unexpected panic attacks.

Antidepressants

DRUG	DOSE (mg/d)	SEDATION	HYPOTENSION	ANTIMUSCARINIC EFFECTS	SEXUAL DYSFUNCTION	WEIGHT GAIN
SSRIs Fluoxetine	10–80	Negligible	Negligible	Negligible	Considerable	Mild
Fluvoxamine	50–300	Negligible	Negligible	Negligible	Moderate	Moderate
Paroxetine	20–50	Mild	Negligible	Mild	Severe	Moderate
Sertraline	25–100	Negligible	Negligible	Negligible	Moderate	Mild
Citalopram	10–60	Mild	Negligible	Mild	Moderate	Mild
Escitalopram	10–20	Mild	Negligible	Mild	Moderate	Mild
Nefazodone	300–600	Moderate	Moderate	Negligible	Mild	Negligible
TCAs Amitriptyline	25–200	Considerable	Moderate	Considerable	Mild	Considerable
Doxepin	75–150	Moderate	Moderate	Considerable	Mild	Moderate
Imipramine	50–200	Moderate	Considerable	Moderate	Mild	Moderate
Desipramine	100–300	Mild	Mild	Mild	Negligible	Mild
Nortriptyline	50–150	Mild	Mild	Mild	Negligible	Mild
SNRIs Venlafaxine	75–375	Mild	Negligible	Mild	Considerable	Mild
Mirtazapine	15–45	Moderate	Moderate	Mild	Moderate	Considerable
OTHER Bupropion	150–450	Negligible	Negligible	Mild	Negligible	Negligible

76 Antidepressants. Side-effects of SSRIs and TCAs used in the treatment of depression in PD.

Nonmotor features of Parkinson's disease

◇ *Agoraphobia* is anxiety about, or avoidance of, places or situations from which escape might be difficult (or embarrassing).

◇ In *specific phobia*, the anxiety is provoked by exposure to a specific feared object or situation, often leading to avoidance behaviour, while *social phobia* is provoked by exposure to certain types of social or performance situations.

◇ *OCD* is characterized by obsessions (which cause marked anxiety or distress) and/or by compulsions (which serve to neutralize anxiety).

◇ *Posttraumatic stress disorder* is characterized by the re-experiencing of an extremely traumatic event accompanied by symptoms of increased arousal and by avoidance of stimuli associated with the trauma. The symptoms are similar to those of acute stress disorder, but they occur immediately in the aftermath of an extremely traumatic event.

◇ *GAD* is characterized by at least 6 months of persistent anxiety and worry.

◆ Most non-PD studies in the elderly have shown that anxiety disorders are less common than in younger adults. In contrast, anxiety disorders in PD have been found to exceed prevalence rates in the geriatric population, and occurred more frequently than in any other medical illness of comparable disability.

◆ The onset of anxiety in late age in PD, and its higher prevalence compared to the geriatric population and other chronic illnesses, is suggestive that anxiety may be aetiologically related to the neurobiological changes that accompany PD and is not simply a behavioural reaction to chronic disability.

◆ GAD, panic disorder, social phobia, phobic disorder, agoraphobia, and OCD have all been described with PD.

◆ Most studies found no significant difference in PD severity between those with and those without anxiety. Symptoms like panic, flushing, and sweating can be principal nonmotor manifestations during the 'off' state. Moreover, pervading anxiety disorders are reported to occur more often among PD patients who experience 'on'/'off' motor fluctuations and symptoms tend to worsen during the 'off' state.

◆ Thus, anxiety itself can be a manifestation of an 'off' state, or can be worsened by motor fluctuations, or can occur independently of, and even precede, motor manifestations.

◆ Relationship to depression and dementia:
   ◇ One study found that 92% of PD patients with anxiety also had depression and 67% of depressed PD patients carried a diagnosis of anxiety.
   ◇ Another study found depression in combination with panic and/or anxiety occurred more commonly among PD patients compared to healthy spouse controls.
   ◇ While two studies hypothesized that anxiety may be less among demented PD patients, others have found no relationship between the two disorders.

◆ Neurobiology of anxiety in PD:
   ◇ Anxiety in PD may be directly related to dopaminergic deficit or can be the result of imbalance in other neurochemical pathways.
   ◇ The main neurotransmitters implicated in the pathogenesis of anxiety are norepinephrine (NE), serotonin, gamma-aminobutyric acid (GABA), as well as some neuropeptides.
   ◇ PET studies in GAD demonstrated decreased glucose metabolism in basal ganglia. A clinical study demonstrated a strong correlation of anxiety to left body parkinsonism. The same correlation was evident for depressive symptoms.

◆ Treatment. The key to successful management of anxiety in PD is its early recognition. A 'team approach' to treatment is most beneficial.
   ◇ Nonpharmacological management, that includes education, counselling, and stress-reduction strategies, should be an integral part of treatment.
   ◇ Studies on the pharmacological management of anxiety in PD are wanting. PD motor symptoms need to be adequately treated. Although most studies find no correlation between PD disability and incidence of anxiety, for the subset of patients with motor fluctuations, there is a clear correlation of anxiety with the 'off' states.
   ◇ *Benzodiazepines*. The majority of PD patients with anxiety will require anxiolytic therapy in addition to dopaminergic medications. Benzodiazepines can be effective for management of GAD, panic disorders, social phobias, but are not effective in OCD. There is no adverse interaction between benzodiazepines and dopaminergic therapy but the potential additive sedative effect of both agents can lead to escalation of daytime somnolence, disruption of sleep–wake cycle, and falling. Cognitively impaired patients can have worsening of their cognition and are at risk for hallucinations. These agents should be avoided in the elderly.
   ◇ *SSRIs*. These are becoming the preferred agents for management of essentially any type of anxiety. SSRIs have a favourable side-effect profile and limited drug–drug interactions. They are widely used in PD for relief of depression and associated anxiety.
   ◇ Concomitant use of SSRIs and MAOB-Is can lead to the development of 'serotonin syndrome' (SS). Non-selective MAOB-Is are contraindicated in patients taking levodopa due to the risk of hypertensive crisis. Selegiline is a selective MAOB-I and does not have monoamine oxidase-A inhibitory effect at the prescribed doses below 10 mg/day. However, at higher doses it becomes a non-selective monoamine oxidase inhibitor. The selegiline package insert has a warning against the concomitant use of either TCAs or SSRIs due to the potential CNS toxicity such as SS, presenting with alterations of mental

status, motor and autonomic dysfunction. Despite the theoretical concern for increased risk of SS with concomitant use of selegiline and antidepressants, it is a rare phenomenon based on the manufacturer's information and survey of a large group of movement disorder specialists.

◇ There are case reports of motor worsening or new-onset drug-induced parkinsonism in the setting of SSRI use, specifically fluoxetine.

◇ *TCAs* act by blocking noradrenaline and serotonin uptake as well as producing long-term increase in their receptor sensitivity. There is a role for TCAs in the management of PD-related pain and sleep dysfunction, as well as hypersalivation. However, their use in PD is limited by their anticholinergic side-effects. TCAs carry a high risk of causing or worsening confusion.

◇ *Bupropion* is a monocyclic antidepressant with indirect DA properties. The most concerning side-effect of the drug is seizures. Its effect on PD anxiety has not been systematically evaluated but its overall 'stimulating' properties may limit its use.

◇ *Buspirone*, which pharmacologically is related to bupropion, also has DA properties. It can be effective for GAD, but is less likely to help panic or social phobia. In PD, the drug was well tolerated in doses up to 60 mg/day but did not produce either antiparkinsonian or anxiolytic effect. At higher doses (100 mg/day) it caused worsening of motor function and worsening of anxiety.

◇ *Mirtazapine* is a newer antidepressant which acts via indirect enhancement of serotonin 5-HT1 receptors as well as direct inhibition of alpha-2 presynaptic adrenergic receptors. Shown to be effective in GAD, it could potentially be a good treatment option for PD patients with anxiety and sleep dysfunction due to its sedative effect at low doses.

Impulse control disorders and compulsive behaviours

◆ OCD-like behaviours have been recently described in PD. Other compulsive behaviours seen in PD include compulsive shopping, compulsive eating, and hypersexuality (**77**).

◆ Pathological gambling is classified under impulse control disorders in the DSM IV and is characterized by 'failure to resist the impulse to gamble despite personal, family or vocational consequences'. In most reports, the behaviour appears after the onset of PD, more often in the 'on' state, and is more closely associated with DAs than with levodopa. It resolves with AA agents or cessation of anti-PD medications.

◆ Examples of compulsive behaviours are dopamine dysregulation syndrome – where patients consume more levodopa than they actually require – and punding.

◆ Punding was first observed among amphetamine and cocaine abusers but has now been described in PD as well. It is a stereotyped motor behaviour in which there is an intense fascination with repetitive handling and examining of mechanical

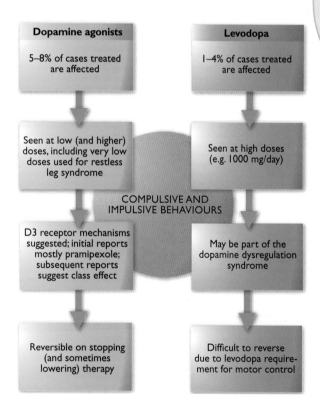

77 Antiparkinson therapy and impulse control disorders. These disorders encompass pathological gambling, hypersexuality, pathological shopping, and pathological eating. A distinction is drawn between the effects of DAs, which can be associated with impulse control disorders from an early stage, and effects of levodopa, which typically occur later in the disease in association with dopamine dysregulation syndrome.

objects, such as picking at oneself or taking apart watches and radios or sorting and arranging of common objects, such as lining up pebbles or rocks. Although punding may be considered a form of compulsion, it is not usually perceived by the patient as relieving a sense of inner tension as is usually the case in OCD. Punding usually occurs after chronic dopaminergic therapy and is relieved by reduction of anti-PD medications.

Sleep disturbances

◆ Several neurotransmitters are involved in sleep–wake functioning: serotonin (dorsal raphe nuclei), acetylcholine (pedunculopontine nucleus), dopamine (striatonigral system, ventral tegmentum, mesocorticolimbic system), and NE (locus coeruleus). There is neuronal loss in the substantia nigra, locus coeruleus, and possibly dorsal raphe nucleus and pedunculopontine nucleus in PD.

◆ Age-related sleep changes include advanced sleep phase syndrome and decreased quality of nocturnal sleep (with increased arousals and awakenings, and daytime naps). The incidence of sleep apnoea and periodic leg movements of sleep (PLMS) is also increased in the elderly.

◆ Other factors contributing to sleep disturbances in PD include: irregular timing of sleep; poor sleep hygiene; physical factors (pain, discomfort, nocturnal akinesia, dyskinesias); cognitive problems (sundowning, nocturnal hallucinations); medication side-effects; and behavioural dysfunction (depression, anxiety) (78).

◆ Sleep complaints have been reported in over 60% of PD patients (79).

Disorders of sleep initiation and maintenance

◆ Characterized by difficulty falling asleep, poor quality of sleep, frequent night-time awakenings, early arousal. Electrophysiologically, there is a reduction in the deep stages of sleep (stages III and IV) and a decrease in REM sleep.

◆ Periodic leg movements of sleep (PLMS).
  ◇ PLMS occur in up to one third of PD patients.
  ◇ Fragmentary myoclonus with irregular myoclonic twitches and jerks of extremities may occur in non-REM sleep.
  ◇ It is still uncertain if the incidence of PLMS is significantly higher in patients with PD as compared to age-matched controls.

◆ Obstructive sleep apnoea (OSA).
  ◇ Although there does not seem to be an increase in the incidence of sleep apnoea in PD patients, there may be an increase in both central and obstructive sleep apnoea in PD patients with significant autonomic dysfunction.
  ◇ OSA has been reported inconsistently in 20–30% of PD patients.

◆ Restless legs syndrome (RLS).
  ◇ Occurs in approximately 20% of the PD population.
  ◇ PD symptoms precede RLS symptoms in 68% of the subjects.
  ◇ DAs, gabapentin, CR levodopa, clonazepam, and opiates are treatment alternatives.

Sleep disturbance	
DISORDERS OF SLEEP INITIATION AND MAINTENANCE	Insomnia Sleep fragmentation (frequent night-time awakenings) Early arousal PLMS Restless legs syndrome Obstructive sleep apnoea
PARASOMNIAS	REM sleep behaviour disorder Nocturnal vocalizations Somnambulism Nightmares Night terrors
EXCESSIVE DAYTIME SLEEPINESS	Medication effect Sudden-onset sleep DBS surgery effect
CONTRIBUTORY COGNITIVE– BEHAVIOURAL DYSFUNCTION	Depression Anxiety Visual hallucinations Dementia

PLMS = periodic leg movements of sleep
REM = rapid eye movements

78 Sleep disturbance. Spectrum of sleep disturbances in PD.

NIGHT

Disorders of sleep initiation and maintenance
Difficulty falling asleep
Poor sleep quality
Frequent wakening
Early arousal

Periodic leg movements of sleep
Myoclonic jerks in non-REM sleep
Restless legs syndrome
Unpleasant or painful sensations
Mainly affects legs but may involve arms
Voluntary movement required for relief
May respond to dopaminergic therapy

REM sleep behaviour disorder
Vigorous physical activity while asleep
Can cause injury to self or others
Represents attempted dream enactment
Muscle tone normally lost when asleep is retained
May predate motor presentation of PD

DAY

Drowsiness and fatigue
Intrinsic to disease
May be a peak-dose effect of dopaminergic medication
Contributed to by depression

Sudden onset of sleep ('sleep attacks')
Described in patients on dopamine agonists
May occur with little or no warning
Obvious implications for driving

79 Sleep disturbance. Sleep complaints are common in PD, with both day and night-time components.

Parasomnias
◆ REM sleep behaviour disorder (RBD) in PD.
  ◇ RBD is characterized by vigorous (and sometimes injurious) behaviour in REM sleep that usually represents attempted dream enactment of vivid, action-filled, violent dreams. The usual loss of muscle tone during REM sleep does not occur in RBD.
  ◇ A study of RBD patients over the age of 50 showed that 11/29 RBD patients developed PD with a mean interval of 3.7 years after RBD diagnosis. It was hypothesized that the pedunculopontine nucleus was a likely site of pathology in combined RBD–PD patients.
  ◇ In another study, RBD preceded the onset of PD in 52% of patients.
  ◇ Low-dose clonazepam (starting with 0.5–1 mg at bedtime) was the most effective drug for the treatment of RBD.
◆ Other behavioural phenomena include: nocturnal vocalizations, somnambulisms, vivid nightmares, and night terrors.

Excessive daytime sleepiness
◆ The reasons for EDS in PD are multifactorial and include: effects of PD motor disability; the disease process; side-effects of dopaminergic medications; co-morbidities (e.g. depression). Even low dosages may be sedating and induce sleep, whereas high dosages may prolong sleep latency and cause sleep disruption.
◆ EDS is found in 15–20% of PD patients compared to 1% of elderly individuals.
◆ The Epworth Sleepiness Scale is a subjective scale widely used in PD sleep studies.
◆ Sudden-onset sleep ('sleep attacks') was first described in nine patients on pramipexole and one patient on ropinirole, causing them to fall asleep while driving leading to accidents. Of these, five patients experienced no warning before the attack. Resolution of symptoms occurred after the medication was discontinued.
◆ On the other hand, appropriate dosages of dopaminergic medication at bedtime may help relieve nocturnal akinesia and rigidity and wearing off symptoms, resulting in improved sleep. One crossover study of 158 PD patients comparing immediate-release levodopa to CR levodopa showed fewer sleep interruptions per night and fewer sleep disturbances with the CR formulation.
◆ A recent study on 10 PD patients with insomnia reported 60% reduction of nocturnal akinesia and complete suppression of axial and early morning dystonia after subthalamic nucleus (STN) deep brain stimulation (DBS). Another study showed seven out of eight PD patients with marked improvement in sleep quality with increased periods of uninterrupted sleep and decreased arousal index.

Effects of cognitive and behavioural dysfunction in sleep
◆ Cognitive and behavioural dysfunction may contribute to sleep problems in PD.
◆ Depression can cause insomnia. In one study, sleep problems were best predicted by the patients' depressive scores.
◆ Sleep disorders are also associated with visual hallucinations. One study showed dementia, age, duration of disease, history of depression, and history of sleep disorder were strongly associated with hallucinations.

◆ Another study comparing 29 PD patients with visual hallucinations to 58 PD nonhallucinators showed a higher incidence of sleep disorders and dementia in the group with hallucinations (22/29 versus 7/58).

◆ A similar study showed that PD patients with visual hallucinations had decreased sleep efficiency, decreased total sleep time, and decreased REM proportion.

Sleep evaluation in PD

◆ Complete history: change of PD symptoms during sleep–wake hours; history of cognitive problems (sundowning, nocturnal hallucinations), motor disturbances (nocturnal akinesia, dyskinesias, painful dystonias), abnormal behaviours (nocturnal vocalizations, nightmares, nocturia, dream enactment, and so on); urinary problems (nocturia).

◆ Sleep diary reflecting hours of sleep, timing of dosage of medications, and so on.

◆ Epworth Sleepiness Scale (ESS) or the Parkinson's Disease Sleep Scale (PDSS) may be helpful (see Chapter 6).

◆ Check for ferritin levels in patients with RLS.

◆ Polysomnographic study: to assess respiratory problems, abnormal movements (RLS, PLMS) and abnormal behaviours (nightmare, night terrors).

◆ Multiple Sleep Latency Test (MSLT) is the considered the gold standard for quantifying EDS.

Management of sleep disorders in PD

◆ Good sleep hygiene with regular sleep–wake hours and regular meal times.

◆ Dopaminergic therapy may need to be reduced if nocturnal dyskinesias are present; increased if nocturnal akinesia is predominant.

◆ CR levodopa may provide added benefit for patients with nocturnal akinesia and early morning worsening of symptoms.

◆ Recognition and treatment of related disorders such as depression, anxiety, psychosis.

◆ For excessive daytime sleepiness or sudden-onset sleep, avoiding or reducing the offending agent (such as DAs) or adding modafinil, methylphenidate, caffeine, dextroamphetamine or similar.

◆ For RLS, DAs, CR levodopa, gabapentin, clonazepam, and opiates are potential treatments.

◆ For PLMS and RBD, low-dose clonazepam is usually helpful.

Autonomic dysfunction

◆ Over the course of PD, more than 90% of patients experience symptoms of autonomic dysfunction, which often results in a negative impact on quality of life.

◆ The pathology of PD has been shown to extend to the autonomic nervous system (**80**). Cell loss and Lewy bodies have been described within the sympathetic system (intermediolateral nucleus of the thoracic cord and sympathetic ganglia), parasympathetic system (dorsal, vagal, and sacral parasympathetic nuclei), and hypothalamus. Lewy bodies have been identified in the oesophageal myenteric plexus of PD patients with dysphagia and were found in the myenteric plexus and submucosal plexuses of the GI tract of 28 out of 30 patients in one study.

◆ PD patients often have a slightly lower resting blood pressure compared to age-matched controls. Orthostatic hypotension is quite common in PD, affecting 20–50% of patients.

◇ It is defined as a drop in systolic blood pressure of >20 mmHg or a decrease in diastolic pressure of >10 mmHg within 3 minutes of standing or head-up tilt. Patients may feel lightheaded and complain of greying vision.

◇ Orally administered levodopa is readily decarboxylated into dopamine and may aggravate orthostatic hypotension.

◇ When orthostatic hypotension is verified, medications that exacerbate the condition (e.g. levodopa, DAs, antihypertensive drugs) must first be reduced or eliminated.

◇ Then, nonpharmacological strategies such as increasing fluid intake, salt, caffeine, support stockings, elevation of legs, and other mechanical measures should be attempted (**81**). If needed, pharmacological agents to raise blood pressure such as fludrocortisone, indomethacin or midodrine may be used (see **82**).

◇ *Midodrine*, an alpha-1 agonist, is usually given three times per day, with the last dose not later than 6 pm to avoid supine hypertension when the patient retires at night. It causes vascular contraction but may inhibit bladder function.

80 Autonomic dysfunction in PD. The sites of cell loss and presence of Lewy bodies on pathological studies are shown. These are common features in PD as it progresses. Some features may predate motor symptoms. Early severe autonomic involvement may indicate MSA rather than PD.

Nonmotor features of Parkinson's disease

Cardiovascular

PD patients have lower resting blood pressure than controls

Orthostatic hypotension affects 20–50%

Systolic drop of 20 mmHg or diastolic drop of 10 mmHg are considered significant

Antihypertensive therapy can often be reduced in PD patients

Gastrointestinal

Sialorrhoea (excess saliva)

Chewing, swallowing, gastric emptying, intestinal motility and defecation may all be slowed

Diarrhoea sometimes occurs as a side-effect of therapy (eg. acetyl-cholinesterase inhibitors, entacapone)

Urogenital

Erectile impotence

Urinary frequency and urgency

Detrusor hyperactivity

Fluid intake should be reduced at night

Bladder medication can assist but may cause prostate-related problems in men

Urodynamic studies are often helpful

Thermoregulatory

Hyperhidrosis (excess sweating) may occur in paroxysms

Cold peripheries and even hypothermia may result from reduced physical activity

---

Autonomic dysfunction: non-pharmacological treatments

SYMPTOM	TREATMENT OPTIONS
ORTHOSTATIC HYPOTENSION	Taper or discontinue unnecessary hypotensive drugs
	Elevate head of bed 10–30°
	Increase dietary salt (add salt tablets)
	Fit thigh-high compression stockings
	Education: avoid standing quickly/ hot environment/straining-type exercises
DYSPHAGIA	Double swallowing, using a 'chin tuck'
	Modify consistency of food
	Adjust timing of medications (e.g. 20–30 minutes before meals)
	Feeding tube placement
CONSTIPATION	Add dietary bulk
	Increase fluid intake
	Take regular exercise
EXCESSIVE DROOLING	Increase voluntary swallowing of saliva
	Suck sugar-free gum or hard candy

◇ *Fludrocortisone*, a mineralocorticoid which works by volume expansion, is an alternative but may lead to pedal or even pulmonary oedema.

◇ *Physostigmine, erythropoietin,* and *octreotide* are reported to be useful but results are still preliminary.

◆ Detrusor hyperactivity occurs in the majority of PD patients. Urinary frequency and urgency are common complaints. It is important to recognize that other factors can contribute to urinary disturbances in the elderly such as benign prostatic hypertrophy. Multiparous women may develop urinary control problems due to pelvic muscle weakness. Urinary symptoms include nocturia, urinary frequency during the day, urinary urgency and urge incontinence. A complete urological evaluation is essential for the correct diagnosis and treatment of voiding problems in DLB.

81 Autonomic dysfunction. Nonpharmacological strategies to alleviate autonomic dysfunction in PD.

Autonomic dysfunction: pharmacological treatments

SYMPTOM	DRUG	DOSE
ORTHOSTATIC HYPOTENSION	Fludrocortisone	0.1 mg daily
	Midodrine	5–10 mg three times per day; last dose should not be after 6 pm to avoid supine hypertension
	Ephedrine	25–50 mg q4–6 hr
	Phenylpropanolamine	
	Ergotamine/caffeine	
	May consider: physostigmine, erythropoietin, or octreotide	
CONSTIPATION	Stool softeners (e.g. docusate sodium)	50–200 mg daily po
	Osmotic laxatives (lactulose, milk of magnesia)	15–30 ml lactulose daily po
	Stimulant laxative (bisacodyl)	10–15 mg po once daily; 10 mg per rectum once daily; or 30 ml fleet enema
	Mineral/tap water enemas	
EXCESSIVE DROOLING	Trihexyphenidyl	2.0–5.0 mg tid
	Benztropine	0.5–1.0 mg tid
	Glycopyrrolate	1.0–2.0 mg tid/qid
	Botulinum toxin type A or B	Injection over parotid and salivary gland
ERECTILE DYSFUNCTION	Sildenafil	50–100 mg 1 hr prior to intercourse; watch for orthostatic hypotension
	Vardenafil	5–20 mg 1 hr prior to intercourse
	Tadalafil	5–20 mg 1 hr prior to intercourse
	Yohimbine	5.0 mg tid
	Papaverine	Intracavernous injection
URINARY FREQUENCY (hyperactive bladder)	Tolterodine	2 mg bid
	Oxybutynin	5 mg tid/qid; patch q3days
	Propantheline	15–30 mg qid
	Hyoscyamine	0.15–0.3 mg qhs–qid
	Imipramine	10–25.0 mg qhs
URINARY RETENTION (hypoactive bladder)	Terazosin	1–10 mg daily
	Doxazosin	1–4 mg daily
	Prazosin	1 mg bid–tid; may increase slowly up to 20 mg/day
	Tamsulosin	0.4–0.8 mg daily
	Bethanechol chloride	10-50 mg po tid–qid; 2.5–5 mg sc tid–qid
PAIN	Minimize 'off' time	Increasing/optimizing dopaminergic medications
	Consider apomorphine	2–10 mg sc with each 'off' state; not more than 10 injections per day

82 Autonomic dysfunction. Pharmacological options for autonomic dysfunction in PD.

◇ Medications often used to treat urinary frequency, urgency and stress incontinence include oxybutynin, TCAs, tolterodine, propantheline, and desmopressin inhaler (**82**).

◇ Most of these drugs should be used cautiously in men with enlarged prostates because of the possibility of bladder outlet obstruction. All have anticholinergic side-effects that may exacerbate cognitive impairment.

◇ Fluid intake should also be reduced at night. A bedside commode may be necessary.

◆ Problems related to the GI system include sialorrhoea, poor motility, changes in appetite, constipation, and weight loss.

◇ Sialorrhoea is more likely the result of decreased swallowing rather than salivary overproduction. Unfortunately, anticholinergic drugs often used to relieve excessive drooling can easily cause confusion and worsen cognitive impairment.

◇ Chewing, swallowing, gastric emptying, intestinal motility, and defecation can all be abnormally slowed. Degeneration of the parasympathetic neurones of the enteric plexus may contribute to poor motility.

◇ GI symptoms such as constipation may not be solely due to autonomic dysfunction. Other factors include: decreased physical activity; diminished intake of food and liquid; reduced force of abdominal muscle contractions; dysfunction of sphincters; and antiparkinsonian medications.

◇ Exercise, muscle conditioning, diet, and medication all help to regulate bowel movement. High-fibre diet plus high-fibre additives, stool softeners, and prune juice should be tried first. If unsuccessful, lactulose can be added. Enemas or laxatives may be used by the third day. Excessive time between bowel movements may call for disimpaction.

◇ If the patient is on a 'pro-cholinergic' medication such as acetylcholinesterase inhibitors, diarrhoea, rather than constipation, may be the issue.

◆ Impotence and other forms of sexual dysfunction are probably underreported in PD. Patients, spouses, and physicians rarely discuss these problems with candour.

◇ There are many potential causes of sexual dysfunction in the elderly, such as vascular insufficiency, prostate enlargement, depression, hormonal conditions (diabetes and thyroid disease), medications (antihistamines, sedatives, antidepressants, antihypertensives), and alcohol use.

◇ A thorough physical examination and urological assessment should be undertaken before treatment is initiated for sexual dysfunction.

◇ The evaluation and treatment of sexual dysfunction in PD can be complex. In addition to medication side-effects (including hypersexuality reported for both levodopa and DAs), depression and poor motor control (nocturnal akinesia) can contribute to decreased libido or impotence. Occasionally, psychotherapy or treatment with the appropriate antidepressant or the addition of levodopa at bedtime may improve symptoms. If not, urological consultation and the use of pharmacological agents such as sildenafil may be considered.

◆ Among the thermal irregularities that may develop in the PD patient, paroxysms of drenching sweats (hyperhidrosis) are the most common, sometimes associated with 'off' states. PD patients may also be susceptible to hypothermia (decrease in body temperature of >2°C) resulting in decreased mentation, encephalopathy, or rigidity and bradykinesia unresponsive to PD medications.

◆ Pain is a common problem in PD, affecting 46% of patients.

◇ Severe rigidity and off-period dystonia are common causes of secondary pain, which is often treated by optimizing dopaminergic medications.

◇ Primary pain is poorly understood but is most commonly seen in the 'off' state. It is usually not responsive to analgesic medications.

◇ Severe pain in the 'off' state can respond quickly to subcutaneous apomorphine.

◆ Olfactory dysfunction.

◇ Most PD patients have a diminished sense of smell. This may precede motor symptoms.

◇ The pathological substrate for PD-related anosmia may be neuronal loss with Lewy body formation in the anterior olfactory nucleus.

Nonmotor features of Parkinson's disease

CHAPTER 6

Motor and nonmotor assessment scales

Motor scales

Unified Parkinson's Disease Rating Scale

◆ The UPDRS is a multimodular scale designed to monitor PD disability and impairment.

◆ Its current version (UPDRS 3.0) is being revised.

◆ It is the most commonly used clinical scale for the evaluation of parkinsonian motor impairment and disability in published treatment trials.

◆ The scale has four sections:
  ◇ Part I — Mentation, behaviour and mood.
  ◇ Part II — Activities of daily living.
  ◇ Part III — Motor.
  ◇ Part IV — Complications of therapy.

◆ Part I examines intellectual impairment, thought disorder, depression, and motivation/initiative (**83**).

UPDRS Part I

	0	1	2	3	4
Intellectual impairment	None	Mild (consistent forgetfulness with partial recollection of events with no other difficulties)	Moderate memory loss with disorientation and moderate difficulty handling complex problems	Severe memory loss with disorientation to time and often place, severe impairment with problems	Severe memory loss with orientation only to person, unable to make judgements or solve problems
Thought disorder	None	Vivid dreaming	'Benign' hallucination with insight retained	Occasional to frequent hallucination or delusions without insight, could interfere with daily activities	Persistent hallucination, delusions, or florid psychosis
Depression	Not present	Periods of sadness or guilt greater than normal, never sustained for more than a few days or a week	Sustained depression for >1 week	Vegetative symptoms (insomnia, anorexia, abulia, weight loss)	Vegetative symptoms with suicidality
Motivation/ initiative	Normal	Less assertive, more passive	Loss of initiative or loss of interest in elective activities	Loss of initiative or disinterest in day-to-day (routine) activities	Withdrawn, complete loss of motivation

83 UPDRS Part I. Mentation, behaviour and mood. Each of four items is scored absent, or at four grades of severity.

◆ Part II evaluates activities of daily living (ADLs)
(**84**).

84 UPDRS Part II. Activities of daily living. Each of 13 items is scored normal or none, or at four grades of severity.

UPDRS Part II

	0	1	2	3	4
Speech	Normal	Mildly affected, no difficulty being understood	Moderately affected, sometimes asked to repeat statements	Severely affected, frequently asked to repeat statements	Unintelligible most of the time
Salivation	Normal	Slight but noticeable increase, may have night-time drooling	Moderately excessive saliva, may have minimal drooling	Marked excess of saliva with some drooling	Marked drooling, requires constant tissue/handkerchief
Swallowing	Normal	Rare choking	Occasional choking	Requires soft food	Requires NG tube or gastrostomy feeding
Handwriting	Normal	Slightly slow or small	Moderately slow or small; all words small but legible	Severely affected, not all words legible	The majority of words are not legible
Cutting food and handling utensils	Normal	Somewhat slow and clumsy, but no help needed	Can cut most foods, although clumsy and slow; some help needed	Food must be cut by someone, but can feed self	Needs to be fed
Dressing	Normal	Somewhat slow, but no help needed	Occasional assistance with buttoning, getting arms in sleeves	Considerable help required, but can do some things alone	Helpless
Hygiene	Normal	Somewhat slow, but no help needed in hygienic care	Needs help to shower or bathe; or very slow in hygienic care	Requires assistance for washing, brushing teeth, combing hair, going to bathroom	Foley catheter or other mechanical aids
Turning in bed and adjusting bed clothes	Normal	Somewhat slow and clumsy, but no help needed	Can turn alone or adjust sheets, but with great difficulty	Can initiate, but not turn or adjust sheets alone	Helpless
Falling (unrelated to freezing)	None	Rare falling	Occasional, less than one per day	Falls an average of once daily	Falls more than once daily
Freezing when walking	None	Rare freezing when walking; may have start hesitation	Occasional freezing when walking	Frequent freezing, occasional falls from freezing	Frequent falls from freezing
Walking	Normal	Mild difficulty, may not swing arms or may tend to drag leg	Moderate difficulty, but requires little or no assistance	Severe disturbance of walking, requiring assistance	Cannot walk at all even with assistance
Tremor (symptomatic complaint of tremor in any part of body)	Absent	Slight and infrequently present	Moderate; bothersome to patient	Severe; interferes with many activities	Marked; interferes with most activities
Sensory complaints related to parkinsonism	None	Occasionally has numbness, tingling, or mild aching	Frequently has numbness, tingling, or aching; not distressing	Frequent painful sensations	Excruciating pain

◆ Part III evaluates motor impairment including speech, facial expression, rest and postural tremor, rigidity, bradykinesia, posture, gait, and postural stability (**85**). This can be used to compare limb features with axial features, upper versus lower body involvement, and right- versus left-sided body involvement.

85 UPDRS Part III. Motor score. This can be scored with the patient in an 'on' state as well as an 'off' state. If only recording one score, specify whether the patient is 'on'. The motor scores relevant to axial symptoms and right and left side of body, as well as upper and lower body involvement, can be calculated (see continuation, next page).

UPDRS Part III

	0	1	2	3	4
Speech	Normal	Slight loss of expression, diction and/or volume	Monotone, slurred but understandable; moderately impaired	Marked impairment, difficult to understand	Unintelligible
Facial expression	Normal	Minimal hypomimia, could be normal 'poker face'	Slight but definitely abnormal diminution of facial expression	Moderate hypomimia; lips parted some of the time	Masked or fixed face with severe or complete loss of facial expression; lips parted >6 mm
Tremor at rest	Absent	Slight and infrequently present	Mild in amplitude and persistent, or moderate in amplitude, but only intermittently present	Moderate in amplitude and present most of the time	Marked in amplitude and present most of the time
Action or postural tremor of hands	Absent	Slight; present with action	Moderate in amplitude, present with action	Moderate in amplitude with posture holding as well as action	Marked in amplitude; interferes with feeding
Rigidity *	Absent	Slight or detectable only when activated by mirror or other movements	Mild to moderate	Marked, but full range of motion easily achieved	Severe, range of motion achieved with difficulty
Finger taps **†	Normal	Mild slowing and/or reduction in amplitude	Moderately impaired; definite and early fatiguing; may have occasional arrests in movement	Severely impaired; frequent hesitation in initiating movements or arrests in ongoing movement	Can barely perform the task
Hand movements ***†					
Rapid alternating movements of hands ****†					
Leg agility *****†					

† Each of these four items is scored according to the same definitions

* Judged on passive movement of major joints with patient relaxed in sitting position. Cogwheeling to be ignored

** Patient taps thumb with index finger in rapid succession

*** Patient opens and closes hands in rapid succession

**** Pronation–supination movements of hands, vertically and horizontally, with as large an amplitude as possible, both hands simultaneously

***** Patient taps heel on the ground in rapid succession, picking up entire leg. Amplitude should be at least 7.5 cm

Motor and nonmotor assessment scales

Continued overleaf

UPDRS Part III continued

	0	1	2	3	4
Arising from chair *	Normal	Slow; or may need more than one attempt	Pushes self up from arms of seat	Tends to fall back and may have to try more than one time, but can get up without help	Unable to arise without help
Posture	Normal erect	Not quite erect, slightly stooped posture; could be normal for older person	Moderately stooped posture, definitely abnormal; can be slightly leaning to one side	Severely stooped posture with kyphosis; can be moderately leaning to one side	Marked flexion with extreme abnormality of posture
Gait	Normal	Walks slowly, may shuffle with short steps, but no festination (hastening steps) or propulsion	Walks with difficulty, but requires little or no assistance; may have some festination, short steps, or propulsion	Severe disturbance of gait, requiring assistance	Cannot walk at all, even with assistance
Postural stability **	Normal	Retropulsion, but recovers unaided	Absence of postural response; would fall if not caught by examiner	Very unstable, tends to lose balance spontaneously	Unable to stand without assistance
Body bradykinesia and hypokinesia ***	None	Minimal slowness, giving movement a deliberate character (could be normal for some persons); possibly reduced amplitude	Mild degree of slowness and poverty of movement which is definitely abnormal; alternatively, some reduced amplitude	Moderate slowness, poverty or small amplitude of movement	Marked slowness, poverty or small amplitude of movement

* Patient attempts to rise from a straight backed chair, with arms folded across chest

** Response to sudden, strong posterior displacement produced by pull on shoulders while patient erect with eyes open and feet slightly apart; (patient is prepared)

*** Combining slowness, hesitancy, decreased arm swing, small amplitude, and poverty of movement in general

UPDRS Part III scoring chart (example)

Speech		2							
Facial expression		2							
Tremor at rest	Face, chin, lips	1	Right arm	0	Right leg	0	Left arm	1	Left leg	0
Action or postural tremor of hands			Right arm	0			Left arm	1	
Rigidity	Neck	1	Right arm	0	Right leg	1	Left arm	0	Left leg	1
Finger taps			Right arm	0			Left arm	0	
Hand movements			Right arm	0			Left arm	0	
Rapid alternating movements of hands			Right arm	0			Left arm	1	
Leg agility					Right leg	0			Left leg	0
Arising from chair		0							
Posture		1							
Gait		1							
Postural stability		0							
Body bradykinesia and hypokinesia		1							

Axial score	Right side score	Left side score

Motor and nonmotor assessment scales

86 UPDRS Part IV. Complications of therapy. These are recorded based on their occurrence within the preceding week.

- Part IV addresses complications of therapy including dyskinesias, clinical fluctuations, and other complications (**86**). Parts I, II, and IV are assessed by interview, part III by physical examination. Parts I to III are scored on a 0 to 4 scale. Part IV is scored using either a rated 0 to 4 scale or dichotomous (yes/no) items.
- Strengths.
  - ◇ It evaluates both motor disability and motor impairment.
  - ◇ There is a UPDRS teaching videotape which helps standardize the application of the motor section, and improves inter-rater reliability (Goetz *et al.*, 1995).
  - ◇ It correlates well with other scales including the Hoehn and Yahr scale, and the Schwab and England scale.
  - ◇ It has good reliability with excellent internal consistency, as well as adequate inter-, and intra-rater reliability.
  - ◇ It has adequate validity, it is sensitive to change in clinical status, and it is responsive to therapeutic actions.
- Limitations.
  - ◇ It is skewed towards motor symptoms, under-representing items such as depression, dementia, psychosis, dyskinesias, and motor fluctuations.
  - ◇ Section I is inadequate for the evaluation of cognition, mood or psychosis in PD.
  - ◇ Section II is culturally biased, as the use of some objects, such as buttons and utensils, is not applicable to all cultures.
  - ◇ Section IV scoring system is different from the other sections, making this information difficult to add together with the rest of the items.
  - ◇ UPDRS does not consider the different co-morbidities that frequently accompany PD.
  - ◇ It does not cover several key elements of PD including anhedonia, bradyphrenia, anxiety, hypersexuality, sleep disorders, fatigue, dysautonomia, and health-related quality of life.

UPDRS Part IV

DYSKINESIAS

Duration
What proportion of the waking day are dyskinesias present?

0	**1**	**2**	**3**	**4**
none	1–25%	26–50%	51–75%	76–100%

Disability
How disabling are the dyskinesias?

0	**1**	**2**	**3**	**4**
not	mildly	moderately	severely	completely

Pain
How painful are the dyskinesias?

0	**1**	**2**	**3**	**4**
not	mildly	moderately	severely	markedly

Presence of early morning dystonia

0	**1**
no	yes

CLINICAL FLUCTUATIONS

Are any 'off' periods predictable as to timing after a dose of medication?

0	**1**
no	yes

Are any 'off' periods unpredictable as to timing after a dose of medication?

0	**1**
no	yes

Do any 'off' periods come on suddenly (e.g. within a few seconds)?

0	**1**
no	yes

What proportion of the waking day is the subject 'off'?

0	**1**	**2**	**3**	**4**
none	1–25%	26–50%	51–75%	76–100%

OTHER

Does the subject have anorexia, nausea or vomiting?

0	**1**
no	yes

Does the subject have any sleep disturbances (e.g. insomnia or hypersomnolescence)?

0	**1**
no	yes

Does the subject have symptomatic orthostasis?

0	**1**
no	yes

Motor and nonmotor assessment scales

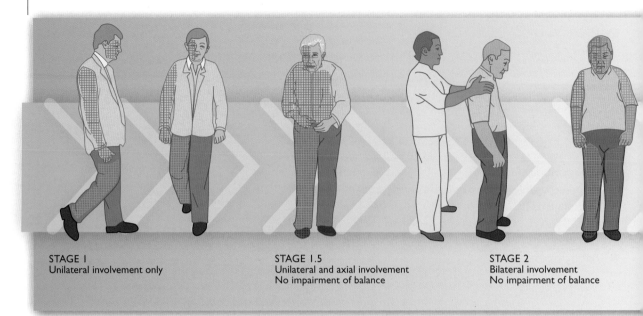

STAGE I
Unilateral involvement only

STAGE 1.5
Unilateral and axial involvement
No impairment of balance

STAGE 2
Bilateral involvement
No impairment of balance

87 **Hoehn and Yahr scale.** Scoring can be readily undertaken on the basis of unilateral or bilateral involvement, and the presence of postural instability.

Hoehn and Yahr (HY) staging scale

◆ It is a descriptive staging instrument designed to estimate function in PD (**87**).

◆ It provides a global assessment of severity of PD based on clinical findings and functional disability.

◆ It was originally proposed in 1967 as a five-point system (1–5), prior to the introduction of levodopa:

◇ Stage I. Unilateral involvement only, usually with minimal or no functional impairment.

◇ Stage II. Bilateral or midline involvement, without impairment of balance.

◇ Stage III. First sign of impaired righting reflexes. Functionally, the patient is somewhat restricted in his activities but may have some work potential, depending upon the type of employment. Patients are physically capable of leading independent lives, and their disability is mild to moderate.

◇ Stage IV. Fully developed, severely disabling disease; the patient is still able to walk and stand unassisted but is markedly incapacitated.

◇ Stage V. Confinement to bed or wheelchair unless aided.

◆ In the early 1990s, a modified version was introduced with half-point increments between stages I and II, and between stages II and III.

◆ Strengths.

◇ The HY scale is the most commonly used instrument to represent severity in PD.

◇ It is easy to apply, brief, and convenient for research and patient care purposes.

◇ It has a strong and consistent correlation with measures of quality of life, motor performance, functional neuroimaging studies, and the UPDRS.

◇ A decline in HY score has prognostic consequences, and can influence therapeutic interventions.

◆ Limitations.

◇ The staging categories are broad, and lump together a large range of impairment severities.

◇ The progression from one category to the next is not linear. Patients may advance from stage I to III without entering stage II, or may begin at stage II without going through stage I.

◇ It strongly favours gait disturbances over other motor symptoms.

◇ There is no teaching material available to help standardize testing.

◇ It scores only motor aspects, and ignores autonomic dysfunction, cognitive decline, behavioural symptoms, and treatment-induced complications.

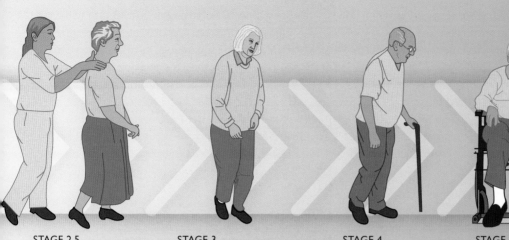

STAGE 2.5
Bilateral involvement with
recovery on retropulsion
(pull test)

STAGE 3
Mild/moderate bilateral involvement
Some postural instability,
but physically independent

STAGE 4
Severe disability but still able
to walk or stand unassisted

STAGE 5
Wheelchair bound or
bedridden unless aided

Schwab and England
Activities of Daily Living Scale

◆ This is a disability scale, with a 10-point descriptive system from complete independence (100%) to complete dependence (0%) (**88**).

◆ It has been extensively used as a standard instrument in PD studies.

◆ Strengths.
  ◇ It is easy to use.
  ◇ It can be completed by the subject, the carer or the physician.
  ◇ It can be used in different chronic neurological conditions.
  ◇ In PD, it can be performed in 'on'/'off' states.
  ◇ It can be used as a measure of quality of life in PD patients.

◆ Limitations.
  ◇ Its validity and reliability have not been established.

88 **Schwab and England scale.** The degree of dependency and assistance required can be categorized according to the parameters shown. Although it is not often done, any number from 0–100% is allowable, e.g. a 75% score would place a patient midway between 70 and 80% in their degree of dependency.

Schwab and England Activities of Daily Living Scale

100%	Completely independent; able to do all chores without slowness, difficulty or impairment; essentially normal; unaware of any difficulty
90%	Completely independent; able to do all chores with some degree of slowness, difficulty and impairment; might take twice as long; beginning to be aware of difficulty
80%	Completely independent in most chores; takes twice as long; conscious of difficulty and slowness
70%	Not completely independent; more difficult with some chores; three to four times as long in some; must spend a large part of the day with chores
60%	Some dependency; can do most chores, but exceedingly slowly and with much effort; errors: some impossible
50%	More dependent; help with half the chores, slower, etc; difficulty with everything
40%	Very dependent; can assist with all chores, but few alone; with effort, now and then does a few chores alone or begins alone
30%	Much help is needed; nothing alone; can be slight help with some chores
20%	Severe invalid; totally dependent; helpless
10%	Complete invalid
0%	Vegetative functions such as swallowing, bladder, and bowel functions are not functioning; bedridden

Motor and nonmotor
assessment scales

Abnormal Involuntary Movement Scale (AIMS)

◆ This is a 12-item instrument originally developed to assess abnormal involuntary movements in psychiatric patients (**89**).

◆ The severity of any involuntary movement (excluding tremor) is scored on a five-point scale (0 = none, 4 = severe) of major muscle groups in the following anatomical regions: orofacial area, extremities, and the trunk. The highest severity observed should be rated.

◆ It includes a global judgement section with two questions directed towards the examiner (severity of abnormal movements, incapacitation due to abnormal movements), and one towards the patient (awareness of abnormal movements).

89 Abnormal Involuntary Movements Scale (AIMS).
Twelve items are used to give a total score. This scoring was designed for assessing neuroleptic therapy, but can be applied to dyskinesia and other involuntary movements in PD.

Abnormal Involuntary Movement Scale (AIMS)

FACIAL AND ORAL MOVEMENTS *

1 **Muscles of facial expression** (e.g. movement of forehead, eyebrows, periorbital area, cheeks; include frowning, blinking, smiling, grimacing)	0	1	2	3	4
2 **Lips and perioral area** (e.g., puckering, pouting, smacking)	0	1	2	3	4
3 **Jaws** (e.g., biting, clenching, chewing, mouth opening, lateral movement)	0	1	2	3	4
4 **Tongue** (rate only increase in movement both in and out of mouth, NOT inability to sustain movement)	0	1	2	3	4

EXTREMITY MOVEMENTS *

5 **Upper** (arms, wrists, hands, fingers). Include choreic movements (i.e., rapid, objectively purposeless, irregular, spontaneous), athetoid movements (i.e., slow, irregular, complex, serpentine). Do NOT include tremor (i.e., repetitive, regular, rhythmic)	0	1	2	3	4
6 **Lower** (legs, knees, ankles, toes) (e.g. lateral knee movement, foot tapping, heel dropping, foot squirming, inversion and eversion of foot)	0	1	2	3	4

TRUNK MOVEMENTS *

7 **Neck, shoulders, hips** (e.g., rocking, twisting, squirming, pelvic gyrations)	0	1	2	3	4

GLOBAL JUDGEMENTS

* 8 Severity of abnormal movements	0	1	2	3	4
* 9 Incapacitation due to abnormal movements	0	1	2	3	4
† 10 Patient's awareness of abnormal movements (rate only patient's report)	0	1	2	3	4

DENTAL STATUS ‡

11 Current problems with teeth and/or dentures	0	1
12 Does patient usually wear dentures?	0	1

* Scored as 0: normal, 1: minimal, 2: mild, 3: moderate. 4: severe
† Scored as 0: no awareness, 1: aware, no distress, 2: aware, mild distress, 3: aware, moderate distress, 4: aware, severe distress
‡ Scored as 0: no, 1: yes

Time	Asleep	OFF	ON without dyskinesia	ON with non-troublesome dyskinesia	ON with troublesome dyskinesia
6:00 am	✓				
6:30 am		✓			
7:00 am				✓	
7:30 am					✓
8:00 am				✓	
8:30 am			✓		
etc.					

- The last two items on the scale assess dental status in a dichotomous (yes/no) fashion.
- It is most commonly used to assess tardive dyskinesia. In patients with PD, the AIMS is used to assess the severity of levodopa-induced dyskinesias.
- Strengths.
  - ◇ This scale is widely used in published studies involving dopamine-blocking drugs and can be used to rate abnormal movements produced by a number of different medical conditions.
  - ◇ It is brief and simple to administer.
  - ◇ It can be easily integrated into a routine clinical examination.
- Limitations.
  - ◇ The amplitude and the frequency of the movements are not rated separately.
  - ◇ There are no guidelines to help standardize scoring between different raters, so inter-rater reliability is dependent upon experience in using the scale.

24-hour motor fluctuation patient diary

- While not a rating scale, the 24-hour diary was developed to assess functional status in PD patients with motor fluctuations and dyskinesias to better target medical and surgical therapies.
- It comprises a 24-hour period, divided into half-hour blocks.
- Patients are instructed to check one of the following clinical states for each half-hour time period: asleep, 'off', 'on' without dyskinesia, 'on' with nontroublesome dyskinesia, or 'on' with troublesome dyskinesia (**90**).
- In the instructions section, a brief and clear definition of each category is given.

90 Parkinson's disease patient diary. This is a sample few hours out of a 24-hour patient-filled diary. The patient is guided to enter their predominant state every half hour and to distinguish components of 'on' to recognize the presence and severity of dyskinesia.

- Strengths.
  - ◇ It is useful to assess 'on' and 'off' time throughout the day, and not at a single point in time, as with the other motor rating scales.
  - ◇ Definitions for each clinical category are specified.
  - ◇ It is simple and easy to complete.
  - ◇ It provides the clinician with a useful method for assessing patient-defined functional status over a period of time.
  - ◇ It is useful both in clinical trials and in day-to-day patient care.
  - ◇ 'On' time with nontroublesome dyskinesias and 'on' time with troublesome dyskinesias correlate well with the patient's perception of good and bad times with regard to motor function.
  - ◇ The diary appears to demonstrate predictive validity and good reliability, and is not influenced by age or gender.
- Limitations.
  - ◇ Diaries are filled out by patients, and thus are subject to patient errors.
  - ◇ Patient compliance appears to decrease after 3 days.

Nonmotor scales

Mini Mental State Examination (MMSE)

◆ This is a standardized and validated scale used as a screening instrument for cognitive impairment.

◆ It measures the following cognitive domains (**91**):

◇ Orientation.

◇ Registration and short-term recall.

◇ Concentration/attention.

◇ Verbal language (naming, repetition, following three-step commands).

◇ Written language (reading and writing).

◇ Visuospatial function (constructing a diagram).

91 Mini Mental State Examination. Various domains of cognitive function are scored up to a maximam total of 30. Although this scoring is not specific to PD the test provides a useful summary of the cognitive performance.

Mini Mental State Examination (MMSE)

ORIENTATION
Patient is asked to name:

Day ☐	Clinic ☐
Date ☐	Floor ☐
Month ☐	City ☐
Season ☐	District ☐
Year ☐	Country ☐ ☐ /10

REGISTRATION
Examiner names three objects; patient is asked to repeat until learnt; six trials allowed

Plant ☐   Key ☐   Ball ☐   ☐ /3

ATTENTION & CALCULATION
Patient is asked to count serial 7s backwards from 100, *or* to spell WORLD backwards

93 ☐	D ☐
86 ☐	L ☐
79 ☐	R ☐
72 ☐	O ☐
65 ☐	W ☐ ☐ /5

RECALL
Patient is asked for names of the three items above

Plant ☐   Key ☐   Ball ☐   ☐ /3

LANGUAGE
Patient is asked to do the following:

Naming Give the the name of:	Pencil ☐	Watch ☐
Repetition Repeat phrase 'no ifs, ands or buts'	☐	
Command Take paper in R hand	☐	
Fold in half	☐	
Place on lap/floor	☐	
Reading Read and obey the command: 'Close your eyes'	☐	
Writing Write a sentence	☐	
Drawing Copy drawing of two intersecting pentagons	☐	☐ /9

- The MMSE is scored using a 30-point scale, with one point awarded for each task that is correctly performed.
  - ◇ Scores between 26 and 30 are generally considered normal in the general population.
  - ◇ Scores between 24 and 26 are considered questionable or indicative of very mild impairment.
  - ◇ Scores below 24 are abnormal, with 21–24 indicating mild cognitive impairment, 10–20 indicating moderate cognitive impairment, and <10 indicating severe impairment.
  - ◇ Age- and education-related norms have been published.
- In patients with PD, the mean annual decline on the MMSE is 1 point. In patients with PD and dementia, the mean annual decline is 2.3 points, which is similar to the rate of decline in patients with Alzheimer's disease.
- Strengths.
  - ◇ It takes approximately 10 minutes to administer.
  - ◇ It can be used in multiple settings, including patients' homes, doctors' offices, hospital settings, long-term care facilities.
  - ◇ Clinical and lay personnel can administer this test with little training, and both test–retest and inter-rater reliability are high.
  - ◇ It provides a useful screen of multiple cognitive domains.
  - ◇ It can give a quantitative measurement of cognitive deterioration over a long period of time.
- Limitations.
  - ◇ Some PD patients may not be able to complete all test items. For example, a patient with severe tremor that persists with action may not be able to write or copy a diagram.
  - ◇ Education affects MMSE scores – highly educated patients may score higher while poorly educated patients may score lower than their level of function suggests. This is especially true when testing concentration, where patients either have to perform serial 7's or spell 'WORLD' backwards. (However, there are norms for educational differences.)
  - ◇ It does not adequately measure abilities mediated by subcortical structures such as executive function, which is commonly impaired in PD patients.

- ◇ It is not sensitive enough to pick up mild cognitive changes, should not be used alone to diagnose dementia, and does not distinguish between dementia and depression.

Dementia Rating Scale (DRS)

- This instrument is used to assess dementia in a wide range of neuropsychological conditions.
- It was originally developed to assess change in cognition in patients with dementia, but can be used to screen for dementia.
- The scale is divided into five subsections:
  - ◇ Attention.
  - ◇ Initiation/perseveration.
  - ◇ Construction.
  - ◇ Conceptualization.
  - ◇ Memory.
- The scale takes about 20–30 minutes to complete.
- The maximum score is 144, with one point awarded for each task that is correctly performed.
- In the revised DRS-2, scores can be compared to age- and education-related norms, giving an idea of how the patient performed in relation to other individuals his/her age.
- Strengths.
  - ◇ Compared to the MMSE, the DRS assesses executive function and evaluates visuospatial function in more detail.
  - ◇ The range of scores is wider and can better evaluate changes in cognition over time.
  - ◇ There is a regression that allows conversion of MMSE scores to DRS scores.
  - ◇ There is a validated alternative form of the test, which minimizes practice effects.
  - ◇ It has been validated in patients with PD and is a good screening test of cognitive function in this population.
- Limitations.
  - ◇ Individuals administering the test need to be trained.
  - ◇ The length of administration limits use.
  - ◇ There is no confrontation naming measure, which would help in differentiating PD dementia from Alzheimer's disease.
  - ◇ There are motor tests such as tapping and alternating movements which may be difficult for PD patients to perform.

Motor and nonmotor assessment scales

Geriatric Depression Scale (GDS)

CHOOSE THE BEST ANSWER FOR HOW YOU HAVE FELT OVER THE PAST WEEK:

1	Are you basically satisfied with your life?	Yes	No
2	Have you dropped many of your activities and interests?	Yes	No
3	Do you feel that your life is empty?	Yes	No
4	Do you often get bored?	Yes	No
5	Are you hopeful about the future?	Yes	No
6	Are you bothered by thoughts you can't get out of your head?	Yes	No
7	Are you in good spirits most of the time?	Yes	No
8	Are you afraid that something bad is going to happen to you?	Yes	No
9	Do you feel happy most of the time?	Yes	No
10	Do you often feel helpless?	Yes	No
11	Do you often get restless and fidgety?	Yes	No
12	Do you prefer to stay at home, rather than going out and doing new things?	Yes	No
13	Do you frequently worry about the future?	Yes	No
14	Do you feel you have more problems with memory than most?	Yes	No
15	Do you think it is wonderful to be alive now?	Yes	No
16	Do you often feel downhearted and blue?	Yes	No
17	Do you feel pretty worthless the way you are now?	Yes	No
18	Do you worry a lot about the past?	Yes	No
19	Do you find life very exciting?	Yes	No
20	Is it hard for you to get started on new projects?	Yes	No
21	Do you feel full of energy?	Yes	No
22	Do you feel that your situation is hopeless?	Yes	No
23	Do you think that most people are better off than you are?	Yes	No
24	Do you frequently get upset over little things?	Yes	No
25	Do you frequently feel like crying?	Yes	No
26	Do you have trouble concentrating?	Yes	No
27	Do you enjoy getting up in the morning?	Yes	No
28	Do you prefer to avoid social gatherings?	Yes	No
29	Is it easy for you to make decisions?	Yes	No
30	Is your mind as clear as it used to be?	Yes	No

Motor and nonmotor assessment scales

One point for each item scored
0–9 Normal
10–19 Mild depression
20–30 Severe depression

Geriatric Depression Scale (short version)

CHOOSE THE BEST ANSWER FOR HOW YOU HAVE FELT OVER THE PAST WEEK:

1	Are you basically satisfied with your life?	Yes	No
2	Have you dropped many of your activities and interests?	Yes	No
3	Do you feel that your life is empty?	Yes	No
4	Do you often get bored?	Yes	No
5	Are you in good spirits most of the time?	Yes	No
6	Are you afraid that something bad is going to happen to you?	Yes	No
7	Do you feel happy most of the time?	Yes	No
8	Do you often feel helpless?	Yes	No
9	Do you prefer to stay at home, rather than going out and doing new things?	Yes	No
10	Do you feel you have more problems with memory than most?	Yes	No
11	Do you think it is wonderful to be alive now?	Yes	No
12	Do you feel pretty worthless the way you are now?	Yes	No
13	Do you feel full of energy?	Yes	No
14	Do you feel that your situation is hopeless?	Yes	No
15	Do you think that most people are better off than you are?	Yes	No

One point for each item scored: 0–5 = normal; 5–10 = suggestive of depression; >10 = indicative of depression

Motor and nonmotor assessment scales

Geriatric Depression Scale (GDS)

◆ This is a valid self-report measure designed to assess depressive symptoms in the elderly with high test–retest reliability.

◆ The original version has 30 items (**92**). A short form (15 items) is also available, which correlates highly with the original (**93**).

◆ Originally designed for use with cognitively intact elderly.

◆ Items address affective and ideational features of depression, rather than somatic or vegetative features.

◆ Each question assesses symptoms during the prior week and is answered in a yes/no fashion rather than on a scale.

92 Geriatric Depression Scale. The 30-point version is shown, left. When an item is checked in the purple field, one point is added and the score can be used to grade the patient between normal and severe depression as shown.

93 Geriatric Depression Scale (short version). Answers in the purple field indicate depression. Although differing sensitivities and specificities have been obtained across studies, for clinical purposes a score >5 points is suggestive of depression and should warrant a follow-up interview. Scores >10 are almost always indicative of depression. See also **94**, Hamilton Depression Scale (HAM-D).

◆ Ten of the items score one point if question is answered 'No'. Some examples include:
  ◇ Are you basically satisfied with your life?
  ◇ Are you hopeful about the future?
  ◇ Are you in good spirits most of the time?

◆ For 20 items, a point is added if the question is answered 'Yes'. Examples include:
  ◇ Do you often feel helpless?
  ◇ Do you often feel downhearted and blue?
  ◇ Do you frequently feel like crying?

◆ A score <10 is within normal limits, scores between 10 and 19 indicate mild depressive symptoms, and scores of 20–30 suggest severe depressive symptoms.

◆ Strengths.
  ◇ It is useful in screening for the presence of depression in the elderly population, which includes many patients with PD.
  ◇ It is a self-report scale – no staff are needed to help administer it.
  ◇ It has been translated into several languages.
  ◇ The scale includes very few somatic features, which may be confounding in a patient with PD.
  ◇ It is easy to administer and can take less than 5 minutes to complete.
◆ Limitations.
  ◇ This scale cannot be used to diagnose depression.
  ◇ It has not been specifically validated in the PD population.
  ◇ It may not be a good choice for younger patients because depression may present differently in that population.
  ◇ Scores may not be consistent or reliable in patients with advanced stages of dementia.

Beck Depression Inventory (BDI)

◆ This is a self-rated scale used to measure the severity of depression.
◆ There are 21 items, evaluating key symptoms of depression.
◆ Each item is followed by four statements, rated from 0 to 3. Patients are asked to circle the number by the statement that best describes their symptoms. For example, for the sadness item:
  ◇ 0 = I do not feel sad.
  ◇ 1 = I feel sad some of the time.
  ◇ 2 = I feel sad much of the time.
  ◇ 3 = I am so sad or unhappy that I can't stand it.
◆ The scores for each item are totalled, with a maximum score of 63.
◆ The BDI can be split into two subscales: cognitive–affective and somatic–performance.
◆ Strengths.
  ◇ It is self-administered.
  ◇ No training of staff is necessary for administration.
  ◇ It can be completed in 5–10 minutes and can be used in multiple settings.
  ◇ Ratings have anchor points.
  ◇ It has been validated in the PD population with altered cut-off scores (17 or greater

indicates presence of moderate depression).
  ◇ The revised BDI-II assesses directionality of changes in appetite and sleep disturbance (increased or decreased), unlike the BDI.
  ◇ It is widely used in research studies.
◆ Limitations.
  ◇ The BDI should be paired with an observer-rated scale if used to measure change in severity over time.
  ◇ There are somatic items (i.e. insomnia, fatigability, work difficulty) which may be difficult to separate from the motor dysfunction of PD.
  ◇ The cognitive–affective subscale has not been validated in PD.

Hamilton Rating Scale for Depression (HAM-D)

◆ This is the most utilized rating scale for patients with primary depression (**94**).
◆ It consists of either 17 or 21 items, rated according to the severity of the depression.
◆ Some items are rated on a 0–4 scale (0 = absent and 4 = most severe) while others are rated on a 0–2 scale (0 = absent or none and 2 = severe).
◆ The total score usually consists of the sum of the first 17 items because the additional items (relating to diurnal variation, depersonalization and derealization, paranoia, and obsession) do not measure the severity of the depression itself and are not common symptoms.
◆ It usually takes 20–30 minutes to administer by a trained rater.
◆ Strengths.
  ◇ It is perhaps the most widely used scale in research studies on depression and has been translated into multiple languages.
  ◇ It can be used to diagnose depression in patients with PD.
  ◇ It has high validity and inter-rater reliability.
  ◇ Change in severity can be monitored over time.

94 Hamilton Depression Scale. An interviewer-rated test consisting of 17 (or 21) multiple-choice questions. In general, the higher the score, the more severe the depression.

Hamilton Depression Scale (HAM-D)

	0	1	2	3	4
Depressed mood (sadness, hopelessness, helplessness, worthlessness)	Absent	These feeling states indicated only on questioning	These feeling states spontaneously reported verbally	Communicates feeling states non-verbally, i.e.: facial expression, posture, voice, and weeping	Patient reports virtually only these feeling states in their spontaneous verbal and nonverbal communication
Feelings of guilt	Absent	Self-reproach, feels they have 'let people down'	Ideas of guilt or rumination over past errors or sinful deeds	Present illness is a punishment; delusions of guilt	Hears accusatory or denunciatory voices and/or experiences threatening visual hallucinations
Suicide	Absent	Feels life is not worth living	Wishes he/she were dead or any thoughts of possible death to self	Suicide ideas or gesture	Attempts at suicide
Insomnia: early	No difficulty falling asleep	Complains of occasional difficulty falling asleep, i.e.: more than ½ hour	Complains of nightly difficulty falling asleep		
Insomnia: middle	No difficulty	Patient complains of being restless and disturbed during the night	Waking during the night; gets out of bed		
Insomnia: late	Sleeps until awakened	Waking in early hours of the morning but goes back to sleep	Unable to fall asleep again if gets out of bed		
Work and activities	No difficulty	Thoughts and feelings of incapacity, fatigue or weakness related to activities; work or hobbies	Loss of interest in activities, either directly reported by patient, or indirectly by listlessness, indecision and vacillation; feels he/she has to push self to work or activities	Decrease in actual time spent in activities or decrease in productivity	Stopped working because of present illness
Retardation (slowness of thought and speech; reduced concentration and motor activity)	Normal speech and thought	Slight retardation at interview	Interview difficult	Obvious retardation at interview	Complete stupor
Agitation	None	Fidgetiness	Playing with hands, hair, etc.	Moving about, cannot sit still	Hand wringing, nail biting, hair pulling, biting of lips
Anxiety: psychological	No difficulty	Some tension and irritability	Worrying about minor matters	Apprehensive attitude apparent in face or speech	Fears expressed without questioning
Anxiety: somatic Symptoms can be gastrointestinal (e.g. indigestion); cardiovascular (e.g. palpitations); respiratory (e.g. hyperventilation); urinary frequency; sweating	Absent	Mild	Moderate	Severe	Incapacitating

Continued overleaf

Motor and nonmotor assessment scales

Hamilton Depression Scale continued

	0	1	2	3	4
Somatic symptoms: gastrointestinal	None	Loss of appetite but continuing to eat; heavy feelings in abdomen	Difficulty eating; requests or requires laxatives or medication for bowels or for GI symptoms		
Somatic symptoms: general	None	Heaviness in limbs, back or head; backaches, headaches, muscle aches; loss of energy; fatigability	Any clear-cut symptom		
Genital symptoms (e.g. loss of libido, menstrual disturbances)	Absent	Mild	Severe		
Hypochondriasis	Not present	Self-absorption (bodily)	Preoccupation with health	Frequent complaints, requests for help, etc.	Hypochondriacal delusions
Loss of weight (either A or B)					
A: by history	No weight loss	Probable weight loss associated with present illness	Definite weight loss (according to patient)		
B: by measurement	<0.5 kg weight loss/wk	>0.5 kg weight loss/wk	>1 kg weight loss/wk		
Insight	Acknowledges being depressed and ill	Acknowledges illness but attributes to bad food, climate, overwork, virus, need for a rest	Denies being ill at all		

◆ Limitations.
◇ There is a heavy emphasis on somatic symptoms of depression, which is confounded in PD.
◇ It takes longer to administer than other rating scales.
◇ It is best suited to individuals with severe illness.
◇ The scale requires significant training and experience to administer.
◇ It is not as useful if the patient has psychiatric symptoms other than depression.

The Brief Psychiatric Rating Scale (BPRS)
◆ This is a standardized scale used for the measurement of significant psychotic and nonpsychotic behavioural symptoms in patients with major mental disorders, mainly schizophrenia (**95**).
◆ There are different versions of the scale but the 18-item scale is the most widely used. It assesses:
◇ Emotional states (anxiety, somatic concern, guilt, suspiciousness).
◇ Cognition (disorientation, conceptual disorganization, and unusual thought content).
◇ Behavioural observations (emotional withdrawal, tension, mannerisms and posturing, grandiosity, depressive mood, hostility, hallucinations, motor retardation, uncooperativeness, blunted affect, excitement).

- Each item is scored on a 1–7 scale where 1 = not present and 7 = extremely severe. 0 means not assessed. Thus, the total score ranges from 18 to 126.
- It takes 15–30 minutes given by a trained rater.
- Strengths.
  - ◇ This is the most widely used and validated psychosis scale for drug treatment in schizophrenia.
  - ◇ It does not require significant training and covers a wide spectrum of behaviours.
  - ◇ It appropriately measures changes with treatment.
  - ◇ It has been used in randomized, controlled drug treatment trials for psychosis in PD.
  - ◇ The scale can be divided into different domains such as 'positive' and 'negative' symptoms.
- Limitations.
  - ◇ It is not a diagnostic tool.
  - ◇ The degrees of severity are not defined so that inter-rater reliability may be low.
  - ◇ It has not been validated in any movement disorder.
  - ◇ PD patients often require a carer in order to appropriately report symptoms.
  - ◇ It is confounded by signs of PD such as akinesia, hypophonia, levodopa dyskinesia, dementia, apathy, and appropriate somatic concern.
  - ◇ The scoring system records a '1' as normal. Since many items are not relevant in PD, changes in single items such as hallucinations or delusions, which are the core features of psychosis in PD, are diluted.
  - ◇ It covers behaviours that are not typically problematic in PD psychosis such as grandiosity, mannerisms, and excitement.
  - ◇ It is not intended for populations with dementia.

Brief Psychiatric Rating Scale (BPRS)

1 SOMATIC CONCERN – preoccupation with physical health, fear of physical illness, hypochondriasis

2 ANXIETY – worry, fear, over-concern for present or future

3 EMOTIONAL WITHDRAWAL – no spontaneous interaction, isolation, deficiency in relating to others

4 CONCEPTUAL DISORGANIZATION – confused, disconnected, disorganized, disrupted

5 GUILT FEELINGS – self-blame, shame, remorse for past

6 TENSION – physical and motor manifestations of nervousness, over-activation, tension

7 MANNERISMS & POSTURING – peculiar, bizarre, unnatural motor behaviour

8 GRANDIOSITY – exaggerated self-opinion, arrogance, conviction of unusual power or abilities

9 DEPRESSIVE MOOD – sorry, sadness, despondency, pessimism

10 HOSTILITY – animosity, contempt, belligerence, disdain for others

11 SUSPICIOUSNESS – mistrust, belief others harbour malicious or discriminatory intent

12 HALLUCINATIONS – perceptions without normal external stimulus correspondence

13 MOTOR RETARDATION – slowed weakened movements or speech, reduced body tone

14 UNCOOPERATIVENESS – resistance, guardedness, rejection of authority

15 UNUSUAL THOUGHT CONTENT – unusual, odd, strange, bizarre thought content

16 BLUNTED AFFECT – reduced emotional tone, reduction in normal intensity of feelings, flatness

17 EXCITEMENT – heightened emotional tone, agitation, increased reactivity

18 DISORIENTATION – confusion or lack of proper association for person, place or time

Each item is scored as follows: 0 = not assessed; 1 = not present; 2 = very mild; 3 = mild; 4 = moderate; 5 = moderately severe; 6 = severe; 7 = extremely severe

Motor and nonmotor assessment scales

95 Brief Psychiatric Rating Scale. The 18 items in the test are rated on seven-point severity scales.

The Neuropsychiatric Inventory (NPI)

◆ The NPI evaluates behavioural abnormalities that occur in demented patients (**96**).

◆ It exists in two forms, one for nursing home residents and one for those at home.

◆ It assesses behaviour in 10 categories. Each is either present, in which case seven or eight

96 Neuropsychiatric Inventory. The scoring is undertaken by the carer rather than the patient and takes account of distress experienced by the carer because of the patient's behaviours.

questions are asked in follow-up, or absent, in which case the next category is assessed.

◆ Scoring is 0–3 in terms of severity and 0–4 for frequency. The severity and frequency scores for each category are then multiplied together and the scores for the categories are added to give a total score. An additional score is obtained for caregiver distress in each category. Severity and frequency are defined to provide relative agreement on scoring across different raters.

◆ Assessment takes 15–30 minutes.

Neuropsychiatric Inventory (NPI)

DELUSIONS	Does the patient believe that others are stealing from him or her, or planning to harm him or her in some way?
HALLUCINATIONS	Does the patient act as if he or she hears voices? Does he or she talk to people who are not there?
AGITATION / AGGRESSION	Is the patient stubborn and resistive to help from others?
DEPRESSION / DYSPHORIA	Does the patient act as if he or she is sad or in low spirits? Does he or she cry?
ANXIETY	Does the patient become upset when separated from you? Does he or she have any other signs of nervousness, such as shortness of breath, sighing, being unable to relax, or feeling excessively tense?
ELATION / EUPHORIA	Does the patient appear to feel too good or act excessively happy?
APATHY / INDIFFERENCE	Does the patient seem less interested in his or her usual activities and in the activities and plans of others?
DISINHIBITION	Does the patient seem to act impulsively? For example, does the patient talk to strangers as if he or she knows them, or does the patient say things that may hurt people's feelings?
IRRITABILITY / LABILITY	Is the patient impatient and cranky? Does he or she have difficulty coping with delays or waiting for planned activities?
MOTOR DISTURBANCE	Does the patient engage in repetitive activities, such as pacing around the house, handling buttons, wrapping string, or doing other things repeatedly?
NIGHT-TIME BEHAVIOURS	Does the patient awaken you during the night, rise too early in the morning, or take excessive naps during the day?
APPETITE / EATING	Has the patient lost or gained weight, or had a change in the food he or she likes?

Answer 'Yes' only if the symptom has been present in the past month, otherwise answer 'No'. For each item answered 'Yes':

Rate the *severity* of the symptom (how it affects the patient)
1 = mild (noticeable, but not a significant change)
2 = moderate (significant, but not a dramatic change)
3 = severe (very marked or prominent; a dramatic change)

Rate the *frequency* of the symptom
1 = occasionally (less than once per week)
2 = often (about once per week)
3 = frequently (several times per week but less than every day)
4 = very frequently (daily or essentially continuously present)

Also, rate the *distress* you experience because of that symptom (how it affects you)
1 = minimal (not very distressing, not a problem to cope with)
2 = mild (slightly distressing, but generally easy to cope with)
3 = moderate (fairly distressing, not easy to cope with)
4 = severe (very distressing, difficult to cope with)
5 = extreme/very severe (extremely distressing, unable to cope with)

- ◆ Strengths.
  - ◇ The training of raters is easy.
  - ◇ There is a teaching videotape available.
  - ◇ The scoring system is clear.
  - ◇ Detailed questions are asked for each category only if the patient endorses problems in that category, which facilitates scoring.
  - ◇ There are different versions for patients living in nursing homes and patients living at home.
  - ◇ Distress of carer is recorded for each category, which helps target treatment.
  - ◇ A comprehensive manual is available from the NPI author.
  - ◇ It is sensitive to changes and is therefore a good tool for intervention studies.
- ◆ Limitations.
  - ◇ Some categories such as appetite/eating, apathy/indifference, and night-time behaviours are confounded by symptoms in PD.
  - ◇ One category, elation/euphoria, is not seen in PD.

Parkinson Psychosis Rating Scale (PPRS)

- ◆ This is the first scale aimed only at measuring psychotic symptoms in PD, and it correlates with other, accepted scales for the measurement of psychosis.
- ◆ Patients are scored 1 (absent) to 4 (severe) on the following six items:
  - ◇ Visual hallucinations.
  - ◇ Illusions and misidentification of persons.
  - ◇ Paranoid ideation.
  - ◇ Sleep disturbances.
  - ◇ Confusion.
  - ◇ Sexual preoccupation.
- ◆ In addition, a Global Functional Impairment score is measured from the carer report.
- ◆ Each severity term is described for each category of symptoms.

- ◆ Strengths.
  - ◇ It does not measure symptoms that may be confounded by the motor dysfunction in PD.
  - ◇ It focuses on three symptoms that are the most common in PD drug-induced psychosis: visual hallucinations, paranoia, and sleep disturbances.
  - ◇ A global scale for functional improvement is included which may be useful for measuring change over time.
  - ◇ Agreement between neurology and psychiatry raters is high.
  - ◇ There is no correlation between PPRS and MMSE scores, indicating that PPRS scores are not influenced by cognitive dysfunction.
- ◆ Limitations.
  - ◇ This test has been evaluated using only a small number of subjects.
  - ◇ One item, sexual preoccupation, is extraneous and not of any value.
  - ◇ Nonvisual hallucinations and nonparanoid delusions are not assessed.
  - ◇ The test is administered to the patient and the carer separately. No instructions are provided for scoring items where the two sources are discrepant.
  - ◇ The global assessment 'moderate' score means 'preoccupied/withdrawn/no motivation', which is frequently seen in nonpsychotic patients with PD, and is usually independent of psychosis.
  - ◇ The category 'illusions and misidentification of persons' is usually seen in nonpsychotic patients with dementia, and is not a typical feature of psychosis in PD.
  - ◇ The category 'sleep disturbances' does not capture the nature of the typical sleep problems of psychotic PD patients. They do not usually have nightmares, but rather have altered sleep cycles and tend to become paranoid at night.

Motor and nonmotor assessment scales

Epworth Sleepiness Scale (ESS)

◆ This is a validated self-report measure of daytime sleepiness covering any designated time period (**97**). It can be used to assess an adult population and has been used in multiple disorders, including PD.

◆ It assesses the likelihood of falling asleep in eight situations common in developed countries (e.g. sitting and reading, watching TV, talking to another person, as a passenger in a car).

◆ Scoring on each item is 0 = would never doze; 1 = slight chance of dozing; 2 = moderate chance of dozing; 3 = high chance of dozing.

◆ Since sleepiness is highly variable and may be normal, the scale assesses sleepiness severity, not pathology. A score >6 is considered indicative of sleepiness; >10 is very sleepy; >16 is dangerously sleepy.

97 Epworth Sleepiness Scale. Different situations where drowsiness or falling asleep may occur are scored.

Epworth Sleepiness Scale (ESS)

Sitting and reading	0	I	2	3
Watching TV	0	I	2	3
Sitting inactive in a public place	0	I	2	3
Being a passenger in a motor vehicle for an hour or more	0	I	2	3
Lying down in the afternoon	0	I	2	3
Sitting and talking to someone	0	I	2	3
Sitting quietly after lunch (no alcohol)	0	I	2	3
Stopped for a few minutes in traffic while driving	0	I	2	3

Each is scored as:
0 = would never doze or sleep
I = slight chance of dozing or sleeping
2 = moderate chance of dozing or sleeping
3 = high chance of dozing or sleeping

◆ Strengths.
  ◇ The ESS is simple, easy to use and takes approximately 2 minutes to complete.
  ◇ It can be self-administered, and questions can be answered by the patient or carer.
  ◇ It is disease independent.
  ◇ It discriminates sleepy from nonsleepy subjects.
  ◇ It is stable over time in healthy people.
  ◇ It changes appropriately with treatment.
◆ Limitations.
  ◇ One question is ambiguous concerning falling asleep at a red light (driver or not driver is not specified).
  ◇ Duration of activities, such as reading and watching TV, is not specified and rapidity of sleep onset is not recorded (falling asleep within 2 minutes of sitting down is different to falling asleep after 30 minutes of reading).
  ◇ The ESS score does not correlate with the multiple sleep latency test, an objective measure of sleepiness.
  ◇ Sleepiness is a variable phenomenon (i.e. medication side-effects, time of day, night's rest), which is not captured by this measure.

Parkinson's Disease Sleep Scale (PDSS)

◆ This gives a visual analogue score for each of 15 features commonly associated with sleep disturbance in PD (**98**) (Chaudhuri *et al.*, 2002). The patient is asked to rate each item based on their experience during the past week, by placing a cross at the appropriate point on the line.
  ◇ Overall quality of night's sleep (item 1).
  ◇ Sleep onset and maintenance insomnia (items 2 and 3).
  ◇ Nocturnal restlessness (items 4 and 5).
  ◇ Nocturnal psychosis (items 6 and 7).
  ◇ Nocturia (items 8 and 9).
  ◇ Nocturnal motor symptoms (items 10–13).
  ◇ Sleep refreshment (item 14).
  ◇ Daytime dozing (item 15).
◆ Strengths.
  ◇ A simple tool for assessing sleep disturbance.
  ◇ Sub-items can detect specific problems, e.g. bladder dysfunction.
◆ Limitations.
  ◇ Zero represents the worse score (opposite to UPDRS scoring).

Parkinson's Disease Sleep Scale

1	The overall quality of your night's sleep is:	AWFUL	EXCELLENT
2	Do you have difficulty falling asleep at night?	ALWAYS	NEVER
3	Do you have difficulty staying asleep?	ALWAYS	NEVER
4	Do you have restlessness of legs or arms at night or in the evening, causing disruption of sleep?	ALWAYS	NEVER
5	Do you fidget in bed?	ALWAYS	NEVER
6	Do you suffer from distressing dreams at night?	ALWAYS	NEVER
7	Do you suffer from distressing hallucinations at night (seeing or hearing things that you are told do not exist)?	ALWAYS	NEVER
8	Do you get up at night to pass urine?	ALWAYS	NEVER
9	Do you have incontinence of urine because you are unable to move due to 'off' symptoms?	ALWAYS	NEVER
10	Do you experience numbness or tingling of your arms or legs which wakes you from sleep at night?	ALWAYS	NEVER
11	Do you have painful muscle cramps of your arms or legs whilst sleeping at night?	ALWAYS	NEVER
12	Do you wake early in the morning with painful posturing of arms or legs?	ALWAYS	NEVER
13	On waking, do you experience tremor?	ALWAYS	NEVER
14	Do you feel tired and sleepy after waking in the morning?	ALWAYS	NEVER
15	Have you unexpectedly fallen asleep during the day?	FREQUENTLY	NEVER

Motor and nonmotor assessment scales

98 Parkinson's Disease Sleep Scale. The patient places a cross on each line in response to the question: 'How would you rate the following, based on your experience in the past week?'. The position on the visual analogue score is converted into a numerical score.

Parkinson's Disease Questionnaire (PDQ-39)

Due to having Parkinson's Disease, how often during the last month have you…

MOBILITY *	0	1	2	3	4
1 Had difficulty doing the leisure activities you would like to do?	☐	☐	☐	☐	☐
2 Had difficulty looking after your home, for example, housework, cooking or gardening?	☐	☐	☐	☐	☐
3 Had difficulty carrying shopping bags?	☐	☐	☐	☐	☐
4 Had problems walking half a mile?	☐	☐	☐	☐	☐
5 Had problems walking 100 yards (approximately one block)?	☐	☐	☐	☐	☐
6 Had problems getting around the house as easily as you would like?	☐	☐	☐	☐	☐
7 Had difficulty getting around in public places?	☐	☐	☐	☐	☐
8 Needed someone else to accompany you when you went out?	☐	☐	☐	☐	☐
9 Felt frightened or worried about falling in public?	☐	☐	☐	☐	☐
10 Been confined to the house more than you would like?	☐	☐	☐	☐	☐

ACTIVITIES OF DAILY LIVING *	0	1	2	3	4
11 Had difficulty washing yourself?	☐	☐	☐	☐	☐
12 Had difficulty dressing yourself?	☐	☐	☐	☐	☐
13 Had problems doing up buttons or shoe laces?	☐	☐	☐	☐	☐
14 Had problems writing clearly?	☐	☐	☐	☐	☐
15 Had difficulty cutting up your food?	☐	☐	☐	☐	☐
16 Had difficulty holding a drink without spilling it?	☐	☐	☐	☐	☐

EMOTIONAL WELL-BEING *	0	1	2	3	4
17 Felt depressed?	☐	☐	☐	☐	☐
18 Felt isolated and lonely?	☐	☐	☐	☐	☐
19 Felt weepy or tearful?	☐	☐	☐	☐	☐
20 Felt angry or bitter?	☐	☐	☐	☐	☐
21 Felt anxious?	☐	☐	☐	☐	☐
22 Felt worried about the future?	☐	☐	☐	☐	☐

STIGMA *	0	1	2	3	4
23 Felt you had to hide your Parkinson's from people?	☐	☐	☐	☐	☐
24 Avoided situations that involved eating or drinking in public?	☐	☐	☐	☐	☐
25 Felt embarrassed in public?	☐	☐	☐	☐	☐
26 Felt worried about other people's reaction to you?	☐	☐	☐	☐	☐

SOCIAL SUPPORT *	0	1	2	3	4
27 Had problems with close personal relationships?	☐	☐	☐	☐	☐
28 Felt you lacked the support you needed from your spouse or partner?	☐	☐	☐	☐	☐
29 Felt you lacked the support you needed from your family or close friends?	☐	☐	☐	☐	☐

PDQ-39 continued

COGNITION *	0	1	2	3	4
30 Unexpectedly fallen asleep during the day?	☐	☐	☐	☐	☐
31 Had problems with your concentration, for example, when reading or watching TV?	☐	☐	☐	☐	☐
32 Felt your memory was failing?	☐	☐	☐	☐	☐
33 Had distressing dreams or hallucinations?	☐	☐	☐	☐	☐

COMMUNICATION *	0	1	2	3	4
34 Had difficulty speaking?	☐	☐	☐	☐	☐
35 Felt unable to communicate effectively?	☐	☐	☐	☐	☐
36 Felt ignored by people?	☐	☐	☐	☐	☐

BODILY DISCOMFORT *	0	1	2	3	4
37 Had painful muscles cramps or spasms?	☐	☐	☐	☐	☐
38 Had aches and pains in your joints or body?	☐	☐	☐	☐	☐
39 Felt uncomfortably hot or cold?	☐	☐	☐	☐	☐

0 = never; 1 = occasionally; 2 = sometimes; 3 = often; 4 = always / unable to do at all

* These headings allow calculation of sub-domains but are not shown to patients

Parkinson's Disease Questionnaire (PDQ-39)

◆ This is a disease-specific measure of subjective health status that is completed by patients.

◆ There are 39 items on the questionnaire (**99**), which give scores that indicate the impact of PD over the past month in eight dimensions of health-related quality of life (**100**):

  ◇ Mobility, ten items.
  ◇ Activities of daily living, six items.
  ◇ Emotional well-being, six items.
  ◇ Stigma, four items.
  ◇ Social support, three items.
  ◇ Cognition, four items.
  ◇ Communication, three items.
  ◇ Bodily discomfort, three items.

◆ Each item can be scored as 0 = never impacts, 1 = rarely impacts, 2 = sometimes impacts, 3 = often impacts, or 4 = always impacts.

◆ Higher scores reflect lower perceived quality of life.

◆ In addition, a global index score, the PD Summary Index (PDSI), gives an overall idea of the impact of PD on health status.

◆ Completion time: 10–20 minutes.

◆ A reduced size questionnaire of only eight items (PDQ-8) shows reasonable correlation with PDQ-39.

99 Parkinson's Disease Questionnaire. The patient completes 39 questions regarding eight aspects of quality of life. Individual domains can be calculated as a sub score (see 100) as well as a PDQ-39 single or summary index score.

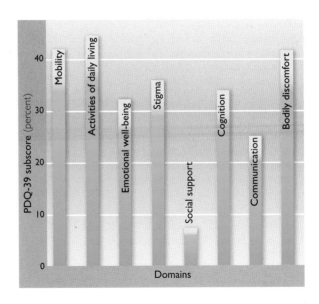

100 PDQ-39 sub scores. The domains are scored from the eight groups of questions, and can be charted as percentages as shown in this example data set.

- ◆ Strengths.
    - ◇ It is the most widely used health-related quality-of-life scale specific for PD.
    - ◇ The questionnaire gives a better idea of function and well-being than motor scales such as the UPDRS or HY.
    - ◇ It has been used to evaluate the efficacy of interventions in clinical trials.
- ◆ Limitations.
    - ◇ It does not include questions specific to fatigue or driving ability, which are important to patients with PD and may impact on their well-being.
    - ◇ It does not address widely prevalent night-time sleep disturbance.
    - ◇ Limited data exist on whether this scale can detect change over time.

Florida Surgical Questionnaire for PD (FLASQ-PD)

- ◆ This is the first assessment tool designed for screening of appropriate DBS (deep brain stimulation) surgical candidates (**101**).
- ◆ There is a five-section questionnaire with questions assessing:
    - ◇ Criteria for the diagnosis of PD.
    - ◇ Potential contraindications to DBS surgery (e.g. abnormal eye movements, abnormal cognitive reflexes, autonomic failure).
    - ◇ General patient characteristics (e.g. age, duration of symptoms).
    - ◇ Favourable/unfavourable characteristics with regard to DBS surgery (e.g. response to levodopa, cognitive function).
    - ◇ Medication trial information subscores.

101 Florida Surgical Questionnaire. A 5-part questionnaire to assess PD surgery candidates, covering diagnosis, contra-indications ('red flags'), clinical characteristics and therapy responses. Sections 3–5 are scored between 0 and 3, with a maximum possible total of 34. The scoring system is designed to assign higher scores to better candidates.

Florida Surgical Questionnaire for Parkinson's Disease (FLASQ-PD)

1 DIAGNOSIS OF IDIOPATHIC PD	No	Yes*
Is bradykinesia present?		
Are **two** or more of the following present? • Rigidity (stiffness in arms, leg, or neck) • 4–6 Hz resting tremor • Postural instability not caused by primary visual, vestibular, cerebellar, proprioceptive dysfunction		
Are **three** or more of the following present? • Unilateral onset • Rest tremor present • Progressive disorder • Persistent asymmetry affecting side of onset most • Excellent response (70–100%) to levodopa • Severe levodopa-induced dyskinesia • Levodopa response for 5 years or more • Clinical course of 5 years or more		

* 'Yes' answers to all three suggest the diagnosis of idiopathic PD

** Any 'red flag' may be a contraindication to surgery

2 POTENTIAL CONTRAINDICATIONS	N/A	Yes**
• Primitive reflexes: presence of a grasp, snout, root, suck, or Myerson's sign (= glabellar tap)		
• Supranuclear gaze palsy present		
• Ideomotor apraxia present		
• Presence of autonomic dysfunction – new severe orthostatic hypotension not due to medications; erectile dysfunction; or other autonomic disturbance within the first year or two of disease onset		
• Wide-based gait present		
• Presence of more than mild dementia – frequently disorientated or severe cognitive difficulties or severe memory problems, or anomia		
• Presence of severe psychosis, refractory to medications		
• History of unresponsiveness to levodopa		
• Parkinsonism is clearly not responsive to levodopa, or patient is dopamine naïve, or patient has not had a trial of levodopa		

FLASQ-PD continued

3 GENERAL PATIENT CHARACTERISTICS	0	1	2	3
Age in years	>80 y	71–80 y	61–70 y	<61 y
Duration of Parkinson's symptoms	≤3 years	4–5 years	>5 years	
On/off fluctuations (medications wear off, fluctuate with dyskinesia and akinesia)	No	Yes		
Dyskinesias	None	<50% of the time	>50% of the time	
Dystonia	None	<50% of the time	>50% of the time	

4 FAVOURABLE / UNFAVOURABLE CHARACTERISTICS				
Gait freezing (if applicable)	Not responsive to levodopa during the best 'on'	Responsive to levodopa during the best 'on'		
Postural instability (if applicable)	Not responsive to levodopa during the best 'on'	Responsive to levodopa during the best 'on'		
Warfarin or other blood thinners	On blood thinner besides antiplatelet therapy	Not on blood thinner besides antiplatelet therapy		
Cognitive function	Memory difficulties or frontal deficits	No signs or symptoms of cognitive dysfunction		
Swallowing function	Frequent choking or aspiration	Occasional choking	Rare choking	No swallowing difficulties
Continence	Incontinent of bowel and bladder	Incontinent of bladder only	No incontinence	
Depression	Severe depression with vegetative symptoms	Treated, moderate depression	Mild depressive symptoms	No depression
Psychosis	Frequent hallucinations	Occasional hallucinations – probably medication-related	No hallucinations	

5 MEDICATION TRIALS				
Historical response to levodopa	Uncertain response, or no trial	History of modest improvement	History of marked improvement	
Trial of Sinemet (carbidopa/levodopa or Madopar or equivalent)	No trial or <3 times a day	Three times a day	Four times a day	>4 times a day
Trial of dopamine agonist	No trial or <3 times a day	Three times a day	Four times a day	>4 times a day
Trial of Sinemet extender	No trial	Trial of either tolcapone or entacapone		
Trial of a combination of Sinemet or equivalent with a dopamine agonist	No trial	Trial of Sinemet or equivalent with a dopamine agonist		

Motor and nonmotor assessment scales

- Higher scores are assigned to better candidates.
- The range of scores is from 0 with 8 red flags (worst possible) to 34 with 0 red flags (best possible).
- Scores of 25 or greater indicate a good candidate for surgery.
- Scores of 15 or below indicate late-stage PD or a parkinsonian syndrome other than PD.
- Strengths.
  - ◇ It is the only tool designed to assess appropriate candidates for DBS surgery.
  - ◇ It is objective and may be useful for non-movement disorders specialists to decide when to refer patients for surgery.
- Limitations.
  - ◇ This scale needs prospective evaluation and validation.
  - ◇ It does not replace the complete multi-disciplinary surgical evaluation.
  - ◇ Some items listed as unfavourable characteristics are controversial (e.g. abnormal cognitive reflexes).
  - ◇ There are certain groups of patients with low FLASQ-PD scores who would still be considered excellent DBS candidates (e.g. patients with treatment-resistant tremor, patients with severe dyskinesias).

Surgical therapy for Parkinson's disease

Surgical options for PD

Surgery can improve symptoms in well-selected patients with Parkinson's disease. While this chapter will be of use to the general practitioner, some sections provide more detailed information for clinicians with particular interest in surgical therapy.

◆ Ablative, or lesion, surgery utilizes a heat probe to destroy small areas of brain tissue. The usual sites are the thalamus (thalamotomy) and the globus pallidus (pallidotomy).

◆ Deep brain stimulation (DBS) is a relatively new, approved procedure that utilizes an implantable device (**102**), which may be used in place of, or in conjunction with lesion surgery.

◇ The DBS device consists of three parts: an implanted pulse generator (IPG), a connecting wire, and a lead – which has four electrode contacts.

◇ The battery-powered IPG is implanted in a subcutaneous pocket below the clavicle. It is connected to the lead via a tunneled extension cable that passes subcutaneously over the clavicle, and across the posterior aspect of the neck and skull.

◇ The lead has four electrode contacts, implanted in a specific area of the brain depending on the disorder. For PD symptoms, the lead may be placed in either the globus pallidus or subthalamic nucleus. Electrical pulses from the IPG interfere with neural activity in the target site.

◇ Each contact can be activated utilizing monopolar or bipolar stimulation, and multiple settings can be adjusted by a neurologist, nurse or trained technician for individual patient needs.

Note: *Much of the material in this chapter was originally published in Chapter 9, 'Key Concepts for Surgical Therapy for Parkinson's Disease and Movement Disorders' in* A Practical Approach to Movement Disorders: Diagnosis and Medical and Surgical Management, *Fernandez et al.,* Demos Medical Publishing, 2007.

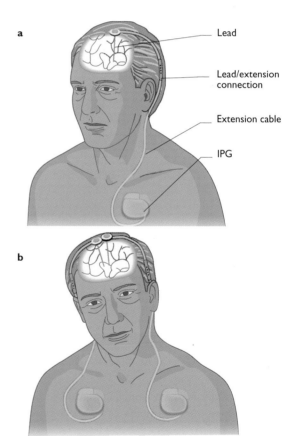

a — Lead

Lead/extension connection

Extension cable

IPG

b

102 Deep brain stimulation. The subcutaneous placement of the pulse generator (IPG) and the position of the connecting wire and lead into the deep brain areas are shown (a). For bilateral DBS (b), two pulse generators are connected to bilateral deep brain stimulators. There is now also a pulse generator that can drive two brain leads from one device.

Selecting candidates for DBS or lesion surgery

◆ Many characteristics are important for ensuring the best possible outcome for DBS (or lesion) surgery in the PD patient.

◆ In general the best candidate profiles include:
  ◇ Idiopathic PD patients who are 'young' with little or no discernible cognitive dysfunction.
  ◇ Those who have undergone multiple medication trials for refractory symptoms.

◆ It is preferable to have patients screened and worked up for PD surgery in an experienced and well staffed multidisciplinary centre because of the complex preoperative, intraoperative, and postoperative care required for these patients.

◆ A simple triage instrument for the general health-care professional/neurologist has been recently published (the FLASQ-PD). This instrument is a survey that can be filled out (in a few minutes) to aid in assessing surgical candidacy, and to assist in picking appropriate candidates for multidisciplinary surgical evaluations. The FLASQ-PD addresses diagnosis, red flags (characteristics making surgery potentially dangerous), favourable and unfavourable characteristics, medication trials, and exceptional circumstances, such as a tremor that will not respond to medication. The instrument allows for a simple score to be awarded that will assess appropriateness of pursuing a full multidisciplinary PD surgical work-up. The scoring scheme is covered in greater detail in Chapter 6 (see **101**).

Age

◆ There is no lower limit on age.
◆ Upper limit on age is usually 75–78 years, but can be modified in select cases (e.g. better physiological age or good overall health may allow criteria to be more flexible).
◆ One study showed a potential increased surgical risk for cognitive dysfunction above the age of 69 (Saint-Cyr *et al.*, 2000).

Diagnosis of idiopathic PD

◆ Patient must meet the diagnostic criteria for idiopathic PD (Brain Bank or other criteria).
◆ Patients should be excluded from surgery if they have another parkinsonian syndrome (PSP, DLB, MSA, including isolated or predominant autonomic type (Shy–Drager), olivopontocerebellar degeneration, or striatonigral degeneration, corticobasal degeneration, vascular parkinsonism, or any other atypical syndrome with parkinsonian features).

'On'/'off' response to levodopa

◆ Patients should be evaluated with a UPDRS after abstaining from their medications the night prior to their surgical candidacy work-up.
◆ Section III of the UPDRS (the motor section) should be performed 'off' medications and then repeated 'on' medications (have them take their medications and wait for them to turn 'on').
◆ The 'on'/'off' percentage difference should (in general) exceed 30% to be a reasonable candidate for surgery.

DBS in PD: perceived outcomes

Does not cure

Bilateral DBS is often required to improve gait, although sometimes unilateral DBS has a marked effect on walking

Smooths out on/off fluctuations

Improves tremor, stiffness (rigidity), bradykinesia and dyskinesia in most cases, but may not completely eliminate them

Never improves symptoms that are unresponsive to your best 'on'. For example, if gait or balance do not improve with best medication response, it is very unlikely to improve with surgery

Programming visits are likely to occur many times during the first 6 months, and then follow-up visits as frequently as every 6 months. There will be multiple adjustments in the stimulator and in the medications

Decreases medications in many, but not all patients

103 Perceived outcomes in DBS surgery. This mnemonic enables discussion with the patient about the benefits and limitations of DBS for PD. *University of Florida.*

Symptoms that respond to surgery (patient education)

- The results of the 'on'/'off' evaluation should be discussed in detail with the patient.
- Only 'motor' symptoms responding to medications are likely to respond to surgery (use the 'on'/'off' evaluation as the guide to discussion).
- If the patient's gait/balance when optimized on their medication and in their best 'on' does not improve, then surgery will probably not help that symptom.
- Nonmotor symptoms like depression, anxiety, and quality of life may improve, worsen, or stay the same, but at this time there are no reliable predictors to discuss with patients.
- It may be useful (both before and after surgery) to have patients study and discuss with their clinican a mnemonic device that may help with perceived outcomes (**103**).

Screening cognitive dysfunction

- It is important to screen for cognitive dysfunction prior to surgery.
- There is no clear definition about what is acceptable cognition to become a surgical candidate.
- Patients who are getting lost or disorientated in general are not good candidates for surgery.
- Patients with moderate to severe frontal and memory dysfunction may not be good candidates.
- Patients with an MMSE score of <26, or a Mattis DRS <116 in general may not be good candidates for surgery.
- It is recommended that neuropsychological testing be done prior to surgery. A typical neuropsychological battery is shown in **104**.
- The neuropsychological screening may need to be repeated after surgery especially if cognitive decline is apparent (it is useful to have baseline testing for comparison in this situation).

Psychiatric screening

- There have been increasing reports of psychiatric complications of DBS surgery.
- These have included but are not limited to depression, depressive symptoms, anxiety, suicide, impulsivity, obsessive compulsive symptoms, aggression, anger, and mania.
- Although preoperative screening is not required, many centres perform it routinely.

Neuropsychological screening tests for DBS surgery

GENERAL	Mini-Mental State Examination (MMSE) Mattis Dementia Rating Scale Wechsler Adult Intelligence Scale (WAIS) III *(information, vocabulary, matrix)*
LEARNING & MEMORY	Paced Auditory Serial Addition Test (PASAT) WAIS III *(Digit forward and backwards)* Hopkins Verbal Learning Task Wechsler Memory Scale (WMS) III *(stories)* Brief Visual Motor Test (BVMT)-R
LANGUAGE	Wide Range Achievement Test (WRAT) III Wechsler Test of Adult Reading (WTAR) Boston Naming Test Controlled Oral Word Association (COWA)
VISUOSPATIAL	Judgement of Line Orientation Test (JOLO) Face Recognition Test
EXECUTIVE	Stroop Test Trail making test *(Trails A and B)* WAIS III *(digit symbols)*
MOOD	Geriatric Depression Scale Beck Depression Scale State-Trait Anxiety Index Visual Analog Mood Scale

104 Neuropsychological screening tests for DBS surgery. This chart is a sample screening used at the University of Florida, but such tests may vary from institution to institution.

- A preoperative screening with a psychiatrist who can perform a structured clinical interview, make preoperative DSM diagnoses, and carefully evaluate depression, anxiety, and mania is useful.
- The psychiatrist may also recommend augmenting the treatment strategy prior to surgery in order to combat depression or anxiety that may impact on the intraoperative procedure and/or outcome.

Special circumstances

- There are circumstances where a patient may not otherwise be a candidate for PD surgery (levodopa 'on'/'off' change <30%, cognitive problems, and so on), but may have a 'special' circumstance (e.g. refractory tremor or dyskinesia).

Surgical therapy for Parkinson's disease

◆ You may consider surgery in the following circumstances, although it may be higher risk:

◇ Medication-refractory tremor.

◇ Medication-refractory severe dyskinesia.

◇ If the patient is on coumadin (warfarin) or other blood thinners (may have to hospitalize and use heparin before and after surgery prior to reinstitution of coumadin (warfarin) depending on individual circumstances).

◇ Medication-refractory and painful dystonia.

Medication trials and optimization

◆ A good medication and optimization trial should be implemented before scheduling PD surgery.

◆ After a patient undergoes PD surgery it will be necessary to optimize medications both in preoperative and postoperative management.

◆ A minority of patients will choose not to have surgery after medication optimization (this should be kept in mind when considering 'staging' the surgery, i.e. do the right side and see if they need the left and vice versa).

◆ Patients should be tried on maximally tolerated doses of carbidopa/levodopa, DAs and dopamine extenders (COMT inhibitors) prior to surgery.

◆ If patients have dyskinesia, 100 mg one to four times a day of amantadine may be useful. If the dose is too high for an individual patient a paediatric elixir is available and can be titrated to effect (but do not use amantadine with patients who have poor kidney function).

◆ For patients with nausea as a result of carbidopa/levodopa consider adding extra carbidopa (25–100 mg) with each dose of carbidopa/levodopa (USA) or adding domperidone 10–20 mg tid (Europe).

◆ For patients with medication-refractory tremor, you may try anticholinergics such as trihexyphenidyl (USA/Europe) or ethopropazine hydrochloride (USA only) – watch for side-effects of mental clouding, urinary retention, confusion.

◆ For patients who are wearing off between medication doses consider switching to regular release carbidopa/levodopa and shortening intervals to every 2, 3, or 4 hours, depending on the situation.

◆ Sudden 'offs' may be treated with ½–1 tablet of carbidopa/levodopa 25/100 mg crushed and in orange juice, or alternatively with dissolvable carbidopa/levodopa tablets or apomorphine.

◆ Dyskinesias and 'on'/'off' fluctuations can often be managed by changing to regular release carbidopa/levodopa, decreasing the dose, and moving medication intervals closer together. Further, DAs (often in lower dose) and dopamine extenders given along with each dose of carbidopa/levodopa may be helpful.

◆ Rarely liquid sinemet (co-careldopa) may be utilized. If liquid sinemet is used one technique is to crush (10) 25/100 mg tablets and put into 1 L of ginger ale, along with a crushed vitamin C tablet. Every mL equals 1 mg of levodopa. Patients can titrate themselves by sipping the potion all day in an attempt to stay 'on' (store away from the sunlight and mix a new batch each day).

Seeing a movement disorders neurologist

◆ Because of the complexity of the screening, it may be beneficial to refer patients to a fellowship trained movement disorders neurologist who is a member of a multidisciplinary and experienced DBS surgery team.

Factors which may improve the success of PD surgery

◆ The following factors which may improve the success of PD surgery for a patient are not evidence based, but are reasonable practice parameters.

◇ Look for well trained multidisciplinary experienced DBS teams.

◇ Look for good (preferably fellowship trained) neurologist–neurosurgeon teams.

◇ Look for a trained neurologist and/or physiologist in the operating room.

◇ Look for a full-time DBS programmer.

◇ Make sure centres perform neuropsychological and, in select cases, psychiatric screening.

◇ Centres should be chosen that will partner with the patient's doctor after the surgery so that medication and programming issues can be addressed efficiently. These centres will help to ensure local follow-up for patients travelling to remote centres for their DBS devices.

Choosing a type of surgery and target site

◆ Both DBS and lesion therapy are effective for the treatment of PD.

◆ DBS is preferred by more patients because it is reversible, and it can be implanted bilaterally without bulbar and cognitive side-effects.

◆ Lesions are preferred by patients who do not want or alternatively cannot have an indwelling piece of hardware. Lesions may also be preferred by those who may not be good candidates for DBS for other reasons (e.g. immunocompromised patients).

◆ Lesions can be performed bilaterally in the subthalamus, and unilaterally in the globus pallidus interna (GPi). Bilateral lesions can be performed in the pallidum, but carry a high risk of side-effects. Thalamic lesions are rarely used in PD because they are limited to tremor control, but bilateral thalamic lesions also may lead to side-effects.

◆ Lesions can be useful in cases where patients do not have access to DBS programming.

◆ The thalamic target is generally effective for tremor, but not the other cardinal manifestations of PD and is therefore not utilized much in PD.

◆ Both the GPi and the STN are very effective targets for DBS therapy (**105**).

◆ It remains unknown at this time which target is better for which kind of patient (symptom profile).

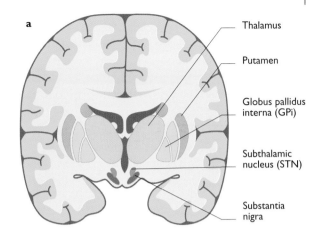

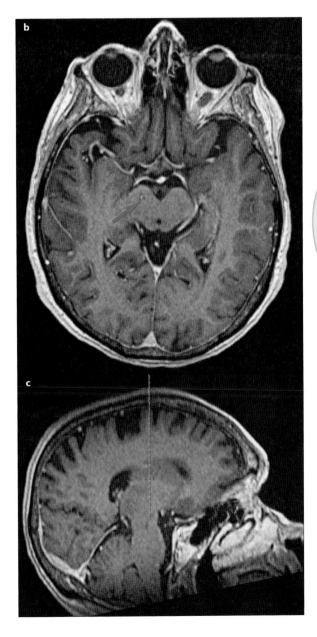

105 Surgical targets for DBS in PD. The main targets used in deep brain surgery are the thalamus, globus pallidus interna and the subthalamic nucleus (a). The thalamus is not commonly a target in PD, but rather for essential tremor. These and other vital structures can be observed on MRI scans. A pre-implantation MRI (b) reveals an axial slice marking the approximate position of the tip of the DBS lead (arrowed), which will ultimately be located in the midbrain below the subthalamic nucleus. A sagittal view (c) reveals the planned trajectory of the DBS lead (dotted line).

Surgical therapy for Parkinson's disease

DBS targeting and lead placement

Stereotactic targeting

◆ High-resolution, volumetric MRI is the imaging study of choice both for preoperative screening and for stereotactic targeting.

◆ The MRI may be obtained after application of an MRI-compatible stereotactic head ring and localizer on the day of surgery, or the MRI may be obtained nonstereotactically prior to the day of surgery and 'fused' to a stereotactic head CT scan on the day of surgery.

◆ The latter approach is advantageous because it saves time and minimizes patient discomfort on the day of surgery and, with appropriate software, the targeting can be performed on the MRI scan in advance of surgery.

◆ Stereotactic targeting is a 'virtual reality' exercise whereby the target and trajectory within the brain are selected in the virtual three-dimensional (3-D) space of the volumetric MRI (or CT, stereotactic ventriculogram, and so on, depending on technique) and translated into the real space of the patient's head using stereotactic reference points or 'fiducials' that exist in both real and virtual spaces (**106**).

◆ In most cases a stereotactic ring is applied to the patient's head under local anaesthesia on the day of surgery.

◆ A CT (or MRI) scan is then obtained with a localizer attached to the ring that allows any point in the volumetric brain image set to be located precisely relative to the position of the ring, which remains in a fixed position relative to the patient's head throughout the procedure.

◆ If an 'image fusion' technique is used, the stereotactic CT is precisely fused to the preoperatively acquired MRI, and targeting is performed on the magnetic resonance images.

Computerized targeting

◆ Computerized 'virtual' targeting generally begins by identifying the patient's anterior and posterior commissures on the MRI and establishing an orthogonal 3-D Cartesian coordinate system with the mid-commissural point as zero.

◆ A standard stereotactic brain atlas is then used to identify the expected location of the selected target.

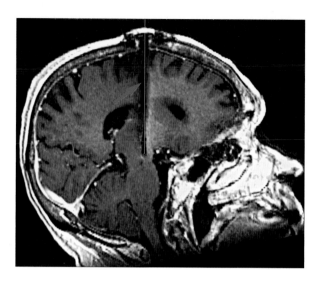

106 Placement of a DBS lead. This sagittal MRI view reveals the track of the DBS lead post-implantation (arrowed).

◆ The target may then be modified based on the images to accommodate for perceived anatomical differences between the patient and the atlas.

◆ Once the anatomical target has been selected, a safe trajectory through the brain is chosen and the 'virtual' operative plan is transferred to the 'real space' of the patient's head using a stereotactic frame that attaches to the head ring during surgery.

◆ The stereotactic coordinates that define the operative target and trajectory from the virtual plan are dialled into the frame, which then guides the implantation of electrodes.

Microelectrode recording

◆ A microelectrode is a recording instrument made of platinum–iridium or tungsten, with a diameter measured in microns, that is used to get close to individual neurones and record their audible activity and physiological characteristics on an oscilloscope.

◆ Microelectrode and/or semi-microelectrode recording allow precise physiological localization of a target region. Each time a new structure is encountered a different physiological signature can be decoded (**107**).

◆ A 3 cm incision is made and an approximately 1.8 cm diameter burr hole is placed in the skull at the stereotactically defined entry site (generally frontal, in the region of the coronal suture).

- Either the lead can be placed at this time by feeding it through the stereotactic guide and the burr hole to the X,Y, and Z coordinates of the anatomically selected target, or the target can be refined physiologically through the use of micro-electrode recording.

- If microelectrode recording is used, the patient is usually kept awake during the operation and minimal to no sedation given (as this may disrupt microelectrode recording).

- The patient's dopaminergic medications are discontinued 12 hours prior to the operation to improve the chances of picking up abnormal physiological activity.

- The authors advocate the use of microelectrode recording, because inaccuracy of stereotactic targeting can be significant and this may lead to a suboptimal outcome or, even worse, unacceptable side-effects.

- The procedure of microelectrode mapping varies somewhat depending on the target. In all cases, however, a 3-D picture of the target structure is constructed and compared to standard atlas slices to determine optimal lead positioning.

- Of course the target in the atlas does not, in general, conform exactly to the same target in a given patient, but the relative sizes and positions of brain structures vary only slightly and an atlas serves as a very useful guide.

107 Microelectrode recording in deep brain areas.
A microelectrode (dotted line) passing through different parts of the brain leaves an electrical signature typical of each area.
Courtesy of Benjamin Walter, M.D. and Jerry Vitek, M.D., PhD.

- Multi-pass microelectrode recording, although potentially more accurate than target verification, is more traumatic.

- Three techniques to perform microelectrode recording are as follows:
  ◇ *1. Target verification.* A microelectrode is inserted and, if the target or enough of the target is encountered, a DBS lead is placed in this location. This technique, although the least traumatic, may be problematic and lead to potentially higher rates of lead misplacement and motor, mood, and cognitive side-effects; it is an issue that is currently under debate.
  ◇ *2. True physiological mapping.* This technique, employed by the authors, involves identifying the physiology of the target and surrounding regions, searching for sensori-motor cells (that respond to movement or touch), identifying borders of the target nucleus with surrounding structures (e.g. optic tract, sensory nucleus, internal capsule), and documenting improvements and side-effects.
  ◇ *3. The 'Ben Gun'.* This involves the use of five simultaneous electrodes and uses stereotactic targeting, physiology, and clinical examination during microstimulation to choose the best location for lead placement.

- The neuropsychological, mood, and behavioural consequences of single or multiple passes with the microelectrode through the frontal lobes and other subcortical structures are currently being researched.

Surgical therapy
for Parkinson's disease

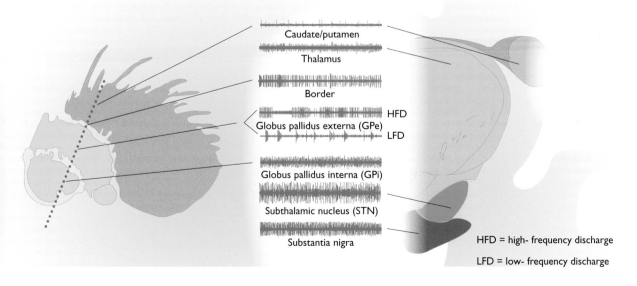

Caudate/putamen

Thalamus

Border

Globus pallidus externa (GPe) HFD / LFD

Globus pallidus interna (GPi)

Subthalamic nucleus (STN)

Substantia nigra

HFD = high- frequency discharge

LFD = low- frequency discharge

Mapping the GPi

- Characteristics that define the GPi region:
  - ◇ Sensori-motor areas are posterior and lateral.
  - ◇ They can be identified by passive manipulations.
  - ◇ The caudal lateral portions of GPi are movement sensitive.
  - ◇ Leg region – medial and dorsal (when compared to arm and face).
  - ◇ Jaw – ventral region.
  - ◇ Anteromedial – nonmotor associative/limbic functions.
- Optic tract location:
  - ◇ Flashing a light into the eyes can give frequency modulation of the background.
  - ◇ Can hear the audio signal.
  - ◇ Can also microstimulate (see speckles of light in the contralateral visual field).
- Internal capsule:
  - ◇ Stimulate at 5-40 microamps (or higher) and 300 Hz.
  - ◇ Stimulation may induce a movement of the limbs or orofacial structures.

Cells encountered while mapping the GPi

- Striatum:
  - ◇ Low spontaneous discharges at 4 Hz.
  - ◇ Injury discharges.
  - ◇ Occasionally tonically active cells at 4–6 Hz.
- Globus pallidus externa:
  - ◇ High-frequency discharges (HFD) (50 ± 21 Hz).
  - ◇ Separated by pauses (high-frequency discharge pause cells).
  - ◇ 10–20% of the cells are low-frequency discharge pause cells (18 ± 12 Hz).
  - ◇ May have high-frequency short-duration bursts.
- GPi:
  - ◇ High frequency (82 ± 24 Hz).
  - ◇ HFD but more tonic.
  - ◇ Also chugging cells: HFDs with pauses that may sound like a chugging train.
  - ◇ 4–6 Hz overt tremor cells can sometimes be heard.

- Border cells:
  - ◇ Frequency (34 ± 19 Hz).
  - ◇ Same as basalis cells, considered aberrantly located basalis cells.
  - ◇ Sound like a motorboat.

Microelectrode localization of the subthalamus

- How much thalamus is recorded prior to entering STN will depend on where the electrode pass is anterior–posterior. Absence of thalamic recording usually indicates a more anterior trajectory has been chosen.
- Cell density in the STN is extremely high.
- Background noise is high and individual cells are difficult to isolate.
- Single neurones discharge at 20–30 Hz, but most recordings are of multiple cells so the apparent discharge frequency is higher.
- As the electrode passes through the inferior border of STN into substantia nigra pars reticulata (SNr) the discharge pattern changes abruptly. Background noise usually dissipates. Single neurones with a higher discharge rate of 50–80 Hz (SNr) can then be heard.
- Important landmarks: medial border STN is lemniscal (sensory) and the lateral and anterior border STN are corticospinal fibres.
- The medial and lateral borders can be defined by microstimulation- and macrostimulation-evoked sensory and motor responses.
- Unlike the GPi target (where the posterior and lateral borders of the initial plane are obtained), the goal of multiple-pass STN mapping is to define the anterior and lateral border.

DBS lead implantation

Macrostimulation

- Once the final target coordinates have been chosen (with or without the use of microelectrode recording), the DBS lead is implanted (or alternatively a lesion is placed).
- The final location of the DBS lead may be verified with intraoperative X-rays (fluorography).
- Macrostimulation is then performed by attaching a temporary pulse generator to the DBS electrode and applying current at each of the four electrode contacts in bipolar configurations.

An intraoperative tester (preferably a neurologist) may rate clinical improvements (tremor, rigidity, bradykinesia, mood changes), or side-effects (muscle contraction due to internal capsule stimulation, paresthesias from stimulation of the sensory thalamus or medial lemniscus, diplopia or visual symptoms from oculomotor or optic tract stimulation, mood changes from stimulation of limbic pathways) to decide if the thresholds for improvement and/or side-effects are acceptable.

The lead may be removed and replaced during this intraoperative session if the intraoperative tester feels the lead is not in an optimal location.

Adjustments (i.e. moving the lead to a different location) of the lead (intraoperatively) after the first macrostimulation pass may lead to current shunts and consequently mislead the intra-operative tester.

The neuropsychological, mood, and behavioural consequences of single or multiple passes with the DBS lead through the frontal lobes and other subcortical structures are unknown.

Securing the lead and implanting generators

After the DBS electrode has been implanted at its final location, it is secured to the skull with a specialized plastic burr hole cover (or alternative securing mechanism) and the redundant electrode is buried under the scalp.

Under anaesthesia, and commonly in a separate, staged procedure, a programmable pulse generator is implanted in a subcutaneous pocket under the clavicle.

An extension cable is then tunnelled under the skin from the pulse generator to the scalp and connected to the implanted electrode to complete the DBS system.

Many centres (including the authors') prefer to wait before attempting to programme the device so that inflammation and brain oedema around the DBS electrode have time to resolve (2–4 weeks).

How long it takes for the neuropsychological, mood, and behavioural consequences resulting from the surgery to resolve remains unknown and under investigation.

DBS programming: general concepts

After activation, the DBS programmer can telemetrically set the device to one of thousands of different stimulation combinations.

The device may be reprogrammed as often as necessary, so stimulation parameters can be adjusted to individual needs.

There may however be trade-offs in programming the stimulator, as the site of optimal motor improvement may cause adverse cognitive or mood side-effects, while a site that does not may also not provide optimal motor control.

It is therefore of paramount importance that the DBS device is in an optimal location. Leads should be implanted into the sensori-motor territories of the target nuclei (e.g. sensori-motor STN, GPi, thalamus), and care should be taken not to place the lead too close to surrounding anatomy that may result in current spread and side-effects.

Leads placed in the nuclei, but causing current spread into limbic and associative regions, may cause further adverse mood and cognitive effects.

Teams implanting and programming DBS devices should monitor the short- and long-term motor, mood, cognitive, and behavioural consequences.

Programming DBS devices

The following simple algorithm can be used in a clinic or GP surgery environment.

◇ Obtain an image and measure placement of the device (CT/MRI or fusion) relative to the anterior commissure, posterior commissure, and midline.

◇ Check impedances (>2000 ohms may be a connection problem, broken lead, or lead fracture; <50 ohms may indicate a short).

◇ Compare the lead location to standard atlas coordinates (see below) as well as your gross impression as to lead placement.

◇ Check impedances of the electrode and perform a battery check.

◇ Use the programmer on monopolar for each lead (0, 1, 2, 3) and (with frequency 135 Hz; pulse width 60–90 ms) slowly increase the voltage until you get a side-effect (preferably not a transient side-effect <30 seconds). Record both the side-effect and the benefit(s) evidenced at each contact.

◇ Choose the best contact in monopolar to use for chronic DBS (remember that voltage used above 3.6 on the Soletra® IPG will dramatically worsen battery life).

◇ Try bipolar settings if DBS has too many side-effects or if you are not satisfied with the benefit.

◇ Slowly decrease the medications and intervals but don't stop them. Look for the best mix of medications and DBS. You may not be able to change many medications with unilateral DBS. Bilateral STN or GPi DBS may require significant medication reductions or changes in medication intervals.

◇ Always programme patients off medications.

◇ Complex patients, after programming is finished, should take their medications and one waits to re-examine them in 'on' medication, 'on' DBS conditions.

◇ Stimulation-induced side-effects may require reductions or changes in both medications and stimulation settings.

◇ If there is great difficulty programming a lead consider referral to an experienced centre as the lead may be misplaced.

Standard coordinates

◆ These are used for estimating lead locations when looking at imaging (atlas approximations).

◆ GPi: lateral 20–21.5 mm; 2–3 mm anterior to mid-commisural point; 4–5 mm inferior to midcommisural point.

◆ STN: lateral 10–12 mm; 0–2 mm posterior to the midcommisural point; 2–3 mm inferior to mid-commisural point.

Side-effects while programming

◆ These help with lead location.

◆ STN DBS: eye deviation, mydriasis, and dizziness (too medial); paraesthesias (too posterior); motor contraction, dysarthria (too anterior and lateral); conjugate eye deviation (too deep); autonomic features (too medial and anterior).

◆ STN DBS may lead to hemiballism, and voltage should be set low and increased slightly over a number of weeks (usually improves with good symptomatic benefit).

◆ GPi DBS: visual symptoms (too deep); motor contraction (too posterior and/or medial).

Postoperative care

◆ A change in skin colour over the impulse generator or the lead could signify infection and patients should go to the hospital immediately for evaluation and/or antibiotics. Infections treated quickly and aggressively may obviate the need for device removal.

◆ Prolonged fever or drainage from the skin close to the device can also signify infection.

◆ Persistent confusion, disorientation, or mental status change can indicate infection, or other neurological emergencies.

◆ Rebound of symptoms can signify lead fractures or battery failure.

◆ Electric shock-like sensations can signify lead shorts.

◆ Sudden excessive spending of money, pressured talking, gambling, or grandiose behaviour can signify mania.

◆ Feelings of doom, dysphoria, crying, and loss of energy may signify depression and should be treated quickly and aggressively because of the potentially increased risk of suicide in DBS patients.

◆ Tenseness, anxiety and anger outbursts can all be the result of DBS.

◆ Persistent postoperative headaches can be a sign of hydrocephalus.

◆ Postoperative seizures can be a sign of haemorrhage, air, or subdural haematomas, and should be followed up with immediate imaging studies.

Risks of DBS

◆ The procedure is expensive, and there are risks beyond the actual surgery, including lead fractures, infections, premature battery failure, and the need for frequent reprogramming.

◆ The surgical risks include infection, haemorrhage, subdural haematoma, stroke, seizure, air embolus, lead misplacement, and hydrocephalus.

◆ The biggest risk is that the results do not meet the patient's preoperative expectations.

◆ Advantages of the DBS system over lesioning therapy include the ability to perform bilateral procedures without speech and cognitive side-effects, reversible effects of stimulation, and the ability to optimize the stimulation parameters for increased benefit.

CHAPTER 8

The role of the nurse practitioner/ physician assistant

Introduction

◆ In the outpatient or clinic setting, the physician assistant (PA) or nurse practitioner (NP) (nurse specialist) obtains a complete history, performs physical examination (**108**), and provides care in collaboration with and under the supervision of a physician. The terms nurse practitioner and nurse specialist can be used interchangeably.

Examining the PD patient

Important elements of the history

◆ Date of diagnosis, and by whom was the diagnosis made. Was it a primary care physician, general neurologist, or movement disorder specialist?

◆ Description of first symptom, and time interval since onset.

◆ Identification of the cardinal features of PD, whether present or absent.

◆ If symptoms are present, identify which side of the body is affected and indicate duration.
  ◇ Tremor.
  ◇ Bradykinesia.
  ◇ Rigidity.
  ◇ Gait or balance difficulty.

◆ Review of PD medications that have been pre-scribed in the past. Key factors include:
  ◇ Duration of therapy.
  ◇ Maximum dose achieved.
  ◇ Regular-release versus CR preparations.
  ◇ Intervals between doses, i.e. 3 hr, 4 hr, tid with meals, and so on.
  ◇ Effectiveness of the medication. For example, did the patient note a slight, moderate, significant, or no noticeable response to dopamin-ergic therapy?

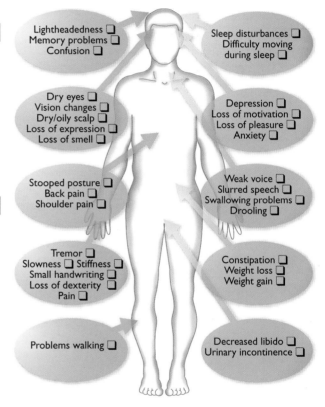

108 Summary of main PD features. The 'Parkin Person' lists the common problems that a PD patient can tick during a clinic visit. *Courtesy of the University at Buffalo Movement Disorders Center.*

  ◇ Side-effects, especially those leading to dis-continuation of therapy, e.g. diarrhoea with COMT-Is, sleep attacks with DAs.
  ◇ Motor fluctuations, including dose failures, delayed 'ons', wearing off, unexpected and/or sudden 'offs', peak dose dyskinesia, diphasic dyskinesia, dystonia.
  ◇ History of treatment with dopamine-blocking agents, including antipsychotic and anti-emetic medications, lithium, reserpine, tetrabenazine.

◆ Most neurologists emphasize the motor aspects of the disease. For completeness, the PA/NP should try to identify possible nonmotor features of PD, such as:
  ◇ Depression.
  ◇ Anxiety and panic attacks.
  ◇ Fatigue.
  ◇ Cognitive problems.
  ◇ Hallucinations, paranoia, and confusion.
  ◇ Sleep disturbance.
  ◇ Sensory symptoms.
  ◇ Constipation and other GI symptoms.
  ◇ Symptomatic orthostasis.
  ◇ Seborrhoeic dermatitis.
  ◇ Urinary frequency, urgency, and nocturia.
  ◇ Erectile dysfunction.
◆ Discussion of social history with particular attention to:
  ◇ Living situation and social support structure: Who is the carer? Does the carer have adequate support? Is respite care available?
  ◇ Where relevant regarding healthcare insurance, knowing the level of cover for prescription medication available from third party payer with regard to prescriptive medications. Knowledge of assistance in terms of co-payment for drugs versus out-of-pocket expense can guide the clinician in therapeutic choices.

Key elements of the physical examination

◆ Orthostatic blood pressure in addition to other vital signs to assess for autonomic dysfunction.
◆ Complete mental status examination with particular attention to frontal lobe function, cognitive function, and praxis to assess for dementia.
◆ Cranial nerve examination, concentrating on vertical gaze to identify other causes of parkinsonism such as PSP.
◆ Deep tendon reflexes. MSA and vascular parkinsonism can present with hyperactive reflexes. Also check for release of primitive reflexes.
◆ Sensory examination, looking for evidence of peripheral neuropathy that could also affect balance.
◆ Motor examination, including performance of part III of the UPDRS.

◆ Observe for spontaneous and/or stimulus-induced myclonus, alien-limb phenomenon, dystonia, dyskinesia, in addition to tremor (rest, posture, and action), bradykinesia, rigidity, and gait. Also assess postural stability.

Parkinsonian syndromes

◆ Consideration of elements in the complete history and physical examination can lead the clinician towards diagnosis of parkinsonian syndromes.
◆ Be aware of the temporal relationship of onset of parkinsonism with concurrent onset of hallucinations, cognitive impairment, fluctuation in mentation, sensitivity to medication. These suggest the diagnosis of DLB.
◆ Dysphagia, orofacial dyskinesia, orthostatic hypotension, constipation, and GI symptoms, laryngeal stridor, hyperreflexia, peripheral neuropathy, axial rigidity, less brisk or unsustained response to levodopa are suggestive of MSA.
◆ History of early falling, difficulty going down stairs, difficulty seeing plate when eating resulting in sloppy eating habits, monotonous speech, 'stone facies' or 'surprised look', pseudobulbar symptoms, and vertical gaze abnormalities are consistent with PSP. Dystonia can also infrequently be seen in PSP patients.
◆ Unilateral dystonia, cortical sensory loss, hand and speech apraxia, myoclonus, asymmetric parkinsonism, and alien-limb phenomenon are found in corticobasal ganglionic degeneration.
◆ Secondary parkinsonism can be caused by medication, infections, vascular insults, and toxins.

Clinical guidance for the PA or NP

◆ The first visit can be quite lengthy. If the diagnosis of PD is made during this visit, be prepared to discuss the implications of the diagnosis.
◆ Explaining that PD is a neurodegenerative disease for which there is no cure can be a bit overwhelming for the patient as well as their family. Stress the fact that there are other conditions and diseases for which there is no cure but for which symptomatic treatment is available, analogous to the symptomatic therapies that are available for treating PD.
  ◇ Two examples are hypertension and diabetes mellitus. Monotherapy may be effective for one person, while combination therapy is indicated for another.

◇ Symptomatic therapy for PD continues to improve, and clinical trials are ongoing. Investigation includes neuroprotective agents as well as symptomatic treatment.
◆ Provide reassurance that progression in PD is measured over months to years, not days to weeks.
◆ Encourage participation in a PD support group, as information regarding the disease is important in living with PD. All information cannot be provided in a single visit.
◆ Encourage activity and exercise. These are elements that can be revisited during future encounters.
◆ Dealing with the difficult patient can be challenging. The value of diplomacy cannot be underestimated. In some interactions, changing from open-ended questions to direct queries may be helpful.
◆ Ask the patient, 'If I were to help you with only one symptom, what is most important to you?' This single question can provide insight into what is most bothersome for this particular person with PD. Physicians sometimes tend to concentrate on the physical examination without asking about the functional state, which is where the PA or NP can be helpful.

Coordinating care

Increasing access to care
◆ Provide dedicated phone number for medical questions for established patients, which is equipped with voice mail.
◇ Outgoing message should identify the PA/NP who will be receiving the call.
◇ Include contact information for new and return patient scheduler, so that misdirected callers can easily reach the administrative staff.
◇ Request that caller state his/her name, spell it, include identifying information such as date of birth, medical record number, or social security number to ensure identification of the proper patient.
◇ Direct caller to include a phone number at which he/she can be reached.
◇ Indicate that if this is an emergency, the patient/carer should call the appropriate services.

◇ Provide timeline for returning calls, e.g. within 24 hours, 2 working days.
◇ Establish dedicated time each day to return calls.
◆ Response to phone calls may include any of the following:
◇ Discussion of symptoms and side-effects.
◇ Adjustments to medications.
◇ Prescription refills. Ask patient to submit requests to the secure fax machine in the pharmacy. Encourage patients to contact their pharmacist or the clinician's office when the last refill is provided. This will reduce the number of last-minute requests.
◇ Referral for appointment for re-evaluation.
◇ Referral to primary care physician or emergency department for non-PD related symptoms.
◆ Consider using e-mail as mode of correspondence with patients, to answer questions quickly. The patient would need to be advised and would need to sign a release for using e-mail.
◆ Depending upon structure of practice, PA or NP can see return and emergency patients.

Providing teaching and education
◆ Basic information regarding diagnosis and progression of disease.
◇ Literature available through APDA (American Parkinson's Disease Association), NPF (National Parkinson's Foundation), UK Parkinson's Disease Society, and European Parkinson's Disease Association can be of great benefit.
◇ For example, APDA currently provides a pamphlet entitled *Hospitalization and the Parkinson's Patient*. Suggest that the patient obtain three copies to be used in the event of an elective surgical procedure or during a hospitalization. One copy should be provided to the physician caring for the patient, one copy is for the nurse, and one remains with the patient and his/her carer.
◆ Medication schedules, titration, and side-effects.
◇ PA/NP in the USA should become knowledgeable about patient assistance programmes for those who do not have prescription medication coverage. Several pharmaceutical companies sponsor such programmes. (See 'Resources', page 161.)

- Support groups and community services.
  - ◇ Have a list of PD support groups within your local area. Provide patients with contact information for the group leader, if not the date, time, and location of meetings.
  - ◇ Compile list of community services including adult daycare services and respite care.
  - ◇ Maintain a list of national organizations for PD and other parkinsonian syndromes and movement disorders for distribution to patients (see Resources section).
- Exercise.
  - ◇ Many PD support groups and retirement communities host PD exercise groups. Encourage participation.
  - ◇ Aquatherapy reduces impact on joints and provides uniform resistance. Swimming also promotes symmetry and is a great form of exercise in the appropriate patient.
  - ◇ Contact local physical therapists and/or fitness centres to see if there are exercise classes available for the PD patient.
- Carer issues.
  - ◇ Question the carer to ensure adequate support is available for allowing time away from responsibility for caring for the loved one with PD.
  - ◇ Contact social worker to determine whether community resources are available for respite care or for at home assistance to provide a break for the carer.
  - ◇ Encourage participation in PD support group. Many groups provide 'break out sessions' for carers, which provide an opportunity to share experiences and learn from others in a similar situation.
- Lifestyle counselling.
  - ◇ Discuss stress reduction.
  - ◇ Discuss ADLs, specifically those which may be impeded or difficult. Suggest assistive devices such as lift chairs when arising from a seated position is extremely difficult, satin sheets when one has problems turning in bed or adjusting the sheets, swivel device for the car when entering or exiting the vehicle is challenging and potentially unsafe.
  - ◇ Provide referral to nutritionist/dietician when indicated.

- ◇ If there are issues requiring assistance, as the stress of coping with a diagnosis of PD and the changes that occur over time can impact on relationships, make referrals to psychologist or counsellor as indicated.
- ◇ Encourage activity. Discuss assistive devices that might enable the person with PD to continue leisure activities he/she enjoys.

Referral to a multidisciplinary team

- Create a directory with contact information for various members of the team which is easily accessible to the PA/NP as well as other staff members.
- Physical therapy for gait and balance training, as well as stretching, range-of-motion exercises.
  - ◇ Consider option of home physical therapy for house-bound PD patients. Identify agencies in the local area, which provide home services.
- Occupational therapy may help, particularly with activities requiring deftness. For example, a person with PD who played the clarinet found benefit from working with occupational therapy.
  - ◇ Make referrals for home occupational/physical therapy safety evaluation to assess the patient's home environment. Therapists can identify any hazards that could contribute to falls, such as throw rugs in doorways and hallways. Therapists also make recommendations for assistive devices, which may be of benefit to the person with PD, as well as the carer.
  - ◇ Assistive devices may include railings, lift chairs, shower chairs, canes, walkers, or wheelchairs.
- Speech and language therapist assessment for evaluation of speech as well as swallow, for patients with hypophonia, dysarthria, or dysphagia.
- Neuropsychology for baseline and annual neuropsychological evaluation.
  - ◇ Patients and family members may find reassurance from normal or minimal impairment.
  - ◇ Neuropsychological evaluation may also help with differentiating PD from parkinsonian syndromes.
  - ◇ In cases where dementia or cognitive impairment is identified, behavioural and/or pharmacological therapy may be initiated.

- Social services.
  - ◇ The outpatient social worker can provide information regarding resources available in the community for respite care as well as home care.
  - ◇ Information regarding financial assistance may also be available.
  - ◇ In cases where placement in an assisted living facility or nursing home may be indicated, the social worker can assist with placement issues, and may also be able to assist the family with obtaining financial assistance for long-term care.
- Psychologist.
  - ◇ The person with PD may need assistance with coping with a diagnosis of PD and the impact of a progressive neurodegenerative disorder on his/her daily life.
  - ◇ The spouse of the PD patient may also be in need of the services of the psychologist, and at times couples' counselling may be indicated.
- Psychiatrist.
  - ◇ Depression, anxiety, and panic attacks are a few of the nonmotor features of PD. Psychiatrists may be in the best position to assist with these particular aspects.
- Driver evaluation. Frequently family members will pose the question of whether the person with PD should be driving. Rehabilitation hospitals typically provide a driver evaluation programme, which includes examination of visual acuity, range of motion, and reaction time. While some programmes offer a driving simulator, others include a road test. The report is returned to the referring clinician as well as to the DMV (Department of Motor Vehicles) (USA) or DVLA (Driver and Vehicle Licensing Agency) (UK).
  - ◇ When requested, the DMV or DVLA may provide a list of driver evaluation programmes.
- Legal professional.
  - ◇ Decisions regarding wills are best made when one is healthy. Encourage patients to consult with appropriate legal professionals to discuss will and testament issues, as well as healthcare surrogate and power of attorney.
  - ◇ Legal professionals may also assist with social security disability/medicare coverage issues as needed.

- Registration personnel.
  - ◇ Ensure that contact information for patient is correct.
  - ◇ Update insurance information.
  - ◇ Provide copies of living will/advance directives. The clinician should also encourage the patient to consider his/her choices for end-of-life issues and discuss them openly with family members.

Specialized services

A number of medications require special initiation and close supervision.

Apomorphine (USA)

- Initiation of apomorphine requires titration in the medical office, which can take up to 3–4 hr. Education and training are provided to the patient and the caregiver (**109**).
- More than one visit may be required for titration.
- The patient presents to the clinic in an 'off' medication state, having discontinued PD medication by 10 pm the evening before the scheduled titration visit.

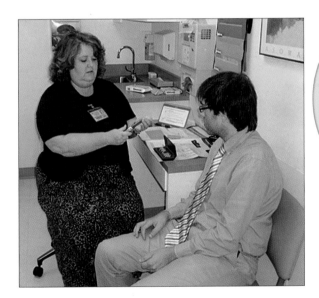

109 Apomorphine titration. A physician assistant educating a young Parkinson patient, who is experiencing motor fluctuations, on how to set up apomorphine injections. In the USA, apomorphine is available as a subcutaneous injection for PD patients experiencing wearing-off episodes, as a 'rescue' therapy. In European countries, apomorphine is available as a continuous subcutaneous infusion.

The role of the nurse practitioner/ physician assistant

Apomorphine titration

FIRST TEST DOSE: 0.2 ML	SECOND TEST DOSE: 0.4 ML Administer at next observed 'off' period, if necessary	THIRD TEST DOSE: 0.3 ML Administer during a separate 'off' period, if second test dose is not tolerated
• Ascertain that the patient is in the 'off' condition	• This dose is administered to the patient who tolerates the 0.2 mL test dose, but does not demonstrate a response. **Do not administer sooner than 2 hrs following initial 0.2 mL test dose**	• Dose of 0.3 mL should be administered to those who do not tolerate the 0.4 mL test dose. **Do not administer sooner than 2 hours following the 0.4 mL test dose**
• Obtain blood pressure (BP) in supine and standing positions prior to dosing.	• Obtain BP in supine and standing positions prior to dosing	• Obtain BP in supine and standing positions prior to dosing
• Patient or carer administers 0.2 mL test dose	• Patient or caregiver administers 0.4 mL test dose	• Patient or carer administers the 0.3 mL test dose
• Obtain BP in supine and standing positions at 20, 40, and 60 minutes following dosing	• Obtain BP in supine and standing positions at 20, 40, and 60 minutes following dosing	• Obtain BP in supine and standing positions at 20, 40, and 60 minutes following dosing
• If the test dose is tolerated, and response is noted, the starting dose should be **0.2 mL**, to be used as needed	• If the 0.4 mL test dose is tolerated, regardless of whether or not there is a response, the starting dose should be **0.3 mL**, used as needed	• If the 0.3 mL test dose is tolerated, the starting dose should be **0.2 mL**, used as needed
• As needed, this starting dose can be titrated upward at increments of 0.1 mL every few days. This can be done on an outpatient basis	• If needed, this dose can be increased in increments of 0.1 mL every few days. This can be done on an outpatient basis. Efficacy and tolerability will need to be assessed from time to time	• If needed, after a few days this dose can be increased to 0.3 mL. This can be done on an outpatient basis. Assess efficacy and tolerability from time to time. The dose in these patients generally should not be increased to 0.4 mL on an outpatient basis
• Those who develop clinically significant orthostatic hypotension with 0.2 mL test dose should not be considered candidates for treatment with apomorphine		

Dose guidance: above volumes are based on the standard available strength in the USA, which is 10 mg/mL. For example, 0.2 mL equates to 2 mg apomorphine. Further dilution of the product (e.g. adding normal saline) or using alternative formulations available in other countries will affect volume and dose equivalences.

110 Apomorphine dosage (USA). Titration of apomorphine to establish patient tolerance.

◆ Confirm the patient in is an 'off' episode.
◆ Evaluate test doses under monitored conditions to determine a dose (0.2 mL, 0.3 mL, or 0.4 mL) that the patient will tolerate (**110**).
◆ Blood pressure is checked before the dose, then 20, 40, and 60 minutes following the dose.
◆ Wait at least 2 hours between doses.
◆ The first test dose is 0.2 mL.

◇ If the patient does not tolerate it, stop.
◇ If the patient tolerates the dose at 0.2 mL and responds, send him/her home on 0.2 mL prn. If needed, the dose may be increased at home by 0.1 mL increments every few days, under the direction of the clinician.

- If the patient tolerates 0.2 mL, but does not respond, then give a test dose of 0.4 mL at the next observed 'off'.
  - ◇ If the test dose of 0.4 mL is tolerated, send the patient home on a starting dose of 0.3 mL. If needed, dose may be increased at home in 0.1 mL increments every few days.
- If the patient does not tolerate 0.4 mL, give a 0.3 mL test dose during a separate, observed 'off' period. If this is tolerated, send patient home on 0.2 mL starting dose. If needed, the dose may be increased at home to 0.3 mL after a few days.
- The maximum recommended dose is 0.6 mL.

Apomorphine (Europe, including the UK)

- A similar approach to that described above is used. Initiation is usually undertaken as a day-case on the ward, following pre-treatment with domperidone 20 mg tid for 3 days.
- Apomorphine is available as a pre-filled syringe with a fixed dilution (5 mg/mL), and also as ampoules which can be diluted with normal saline. For this reason, always check the dose in milligrams rather than considering the dose only in terms of volume (mL).
- Apomorphine is also available in Europe for semi-continuous (i.e. waking day) subcutaneous infusion by a portable battery-powered mini-pump device. Initiation is usually at 1 mg/hr, with increments of 0.5 mg/hr each day, and with maintenance usually between 2 and 6 mg/hr (most typically 3, 3.5 or 4 mg/hr). Oral DAs are usually discontinued and oral levodopa doses are sometimes reduced or even stopped.
- Consult the product summary for more details.

Clozapine

- Clozapine administration initially requires weekly CBC with differential to monitor for agranulocytosis.
- The absolute neutrophil count (ANC) can be calculated by multiplying the total WBC count by the percentage of neutrophils.
- Percentage of neutrophils is the sum of the percentage of segmented neutrophils plus the percentage of band neutrophils.
- Acceptable dispensing values are WBC counts $\geq 3 \times 10^9$/L and ANCs $\geq 1.5 \times 10^9$/L.
- A WBC count $<3.5 \times 10^9$/L or an ANC $<2 \times 10^9$/L is an indication of leucopenia or granulocytopenia, and patients should be monitored closely.

- Frequency of monitoring is based on stage of therapy or results from WBC count and ANC monitoring tests.
- At initiation of therapy, WBC and ANC monitoring is obtained weekly for 6 months as long as haematological values for monitoring are WBC $\geq 3.5 \times 10^9$/L, ANC $\geq 2 \times 10^9$/L.
- If all results for WBC $\geq 3.5 \times 10^9$/L, and ANC $\geq 2 \times 10^9$/L, after 6 months of therapy, monitoring between 6 months and 12 months of therapy can be performed every 2 weeks.
- If all results for WBC $\geq 3.5 \times 10^9$/L and ANC $\geq 2 \times 10^9$/L after 12 months of therapy, monitoring can be extended to every 4 weeks indefinitely.
- At discontinuation of therapy, WBC and ANC monitoring should occur weekly for at least 4 weeks from day of discontinuation or until WBC $\geq 3.5 \times 10^9$/L and ANC $\geq 2 \times 10^9$/L.
- If there is a single drop or cumulative drop within 3 weeks of WBC $\geq 3 \times 10^9$/L or ANC $\geq 1.5 \times 10^9$/L:
  - ◇ Repeat WBC and ANC.
  - ◇ If repeat values are WBC 3–3.5 $\times 10^9$/L and ANC $>2 \times 10^9$/L, then monitor twice weekly.
- If there is mild leucopenia, WBC 3–3.5 $\times 10^9$/L and/or mild granulocytopenia, ANC 1.5–2 $\times 10^9$/L, perform twice-weekly monitoring until WBC $>3.5 \times 10^9$/L and ANC $>2 \times 10^9$/L then return to previous monitoring frequency.
- In cases of moderate leucopenia, WBC 2–3 $\times 10^9$/L and/or moderate granulocytopenia, ANC >1.0–1.5 $\times 10^9$/L:
  - ◇ Interrupt therapy.
  - ◇ Daily monitoring of WBC and ANC until WBC $>3 \times 10^9$/L and ANC $>1.5 \times 10^9$/L.
  - ◇ Twice-weekly monitoring until WBC $>3.5 \times 10^9$/L and ANC $>2 \times 10^9$/L.
  - ◇ May rechallenge when WBC $>3.5 \times 10^9$/L and ANC $>2 \times 10^9$/L.
  - ◇ If rechallenged, monitor weekly for 1 year before returning to the usual monitoring schedule of every 2 weeks for 6 months and then every 4 weeks *ad infinitum*.
- Severe leucopenia, WBC $<2 \times 10^9$/L and/or severe granulocytopenia, ANC $<1.0 \times 10^9$/L:
  - ◇ Discontinue treatment and do not rechallenge patient.
  - ◇ Monitor until normal and for at least 4 weeks from day of discontinuation thus: daily until WBC $>3 \times 10^9$/L and ANC $>1.5 \times 10^9$/L; twice weekly until WBC $>3.5 \times 10^9$/L and ANC $>2 \times 10^9$/L; weekly after WBC $>3.5 \times 10^9$/L.

The role of the nurse practitioner/ physician assistant

◆ Agranulocytosis, ANC <0.5 × 10⁹/L:
 ◇ Discontinue treatment and do not rechallenge patient.
 ◇ Monitor until normal and for at least 4 weeks from discontinuation as follows: daily until WBC >3 × 10⁹/L and ANC >1.5 × 10⁹/L; twice weekly until WBC >3.5 × 10⁹/L and ANC >2 × 10⁹/L; weekly after WBC >3.5 × 10⁹/L.

◆ Do not initiate in patients with a history of myeloproliferative disorder or clozapine-induced agranulocytosis or granulocytopenia.

◆ Above units can be converted to conventional units as follows: 1.0×10^9 cells/L = 1000 cells/mm³.

◆ *Initiation and monitoring of clozapine is only performed through registration with a mandatory monitoring scheme.*

Tolcapone

◆ Tolcapone administration requires baseline serum glutamic-pyruvic transaminase (SGPT/ALT) and serum glutamic-oxaloacetic transaminase (SGOT/AST), with levels checked every month for 6 months and as needed thereafter.

◆ If the dose is increased to 200 mg tid, liver enzyme monitoring should take place before increasing the dose.

◆ Because of the rare possibility of acute fulminant hepatitis with tolcapone, it should not be initiated if the patient exhibits clinical evidence of liver disease or has two SGPT/ALT or SGOT/AST values greater than the upper limit of normal.

◆ Tolcapone should be discontinued if the ALT or AST levels exceed the upper limit of normal or clinical signs or symptoms suggest the onset of hepatic failure (persistent nausea, fatigue, lethargy, anorexia, jaundice, dark urine, pruritus, and right upper quadrant tenderness).

Care of DBS patients

◆ Coordinate referrals to members of the team evaluating potential DBS surgical candidate:
 ◇ Neurosurgeon.
 ◇ Neuropsychologist.
 ◇ Psychiatrist.
 ◇ Radiologist.

◆ Programme the DBS device (**111**):
 ◇ At intervals designated as standard of care.
 ◇ As needed.

◆ PD patients should be programmed in the off medication state. They should be advised to discontinue their medications at 10 pm the night before the visit.

◆ As patients present off medication, it may be best to schedule visits in the morning to reduce the time the individual is in the unmedicated state.

◆ Impedances and battery status should be checked at every office visit.
 ◇ If impedances are abnormal, and the clinician is concerned there may be a lead fracture, send the patient for plain films, including a shunt series and chest film.

◆ Reset the counters at each programming visit.
 ◇ If there are numerous activations since the time of the last visit, inquire as to whether the device has been turned off for any reason.
 ◇ If there have not been deliberate deactivations of the device, question whether the person has been exposed to a magnetic field, which can include freezers as well as security systems in retail stores.

◆ Monitor motor performance in at least two conditions to determine the ideal parameters:
 ◇ Off medication/on stimulation.
 ◇ On medication/on stimulation.

◆ May coordinate follow-up imaging studies for lead localization if needed.

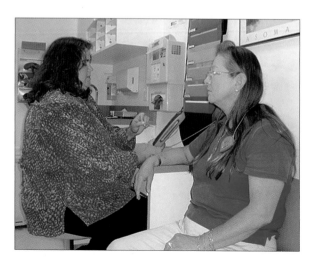

1 1 1 DBS device programming. Finding the optimal settings requires patience and good communication.

CHAPTER 9

The role of the physical and occupational therapist

Movement and functional deficits in the PD patient

◆ The role of the occupational therapist (OT) and the physical therapist (PT) in the treatment of individuals with PD is to address the patient's motor dysfunction in an effort to increase their functional independence.

◆ Dependence in ADLs is one of the primary reasons cited by PD patients and their carers as a reason to seek treatment.

◆ This loss of function is also reported to contribute greatly to a perceived decline in quality of life for these individuals.

Motor symptoms

◆ Functional abilities in PD patients are partially impaired by motor symptoms. The consequences of common motor symptoms displayed are:

◇ Bradykinesia and akinesia often result in difficulty performing purposeful movement. There is greater energy expenditure and patients demonstrate difficulty with simultaneous tasks, such as walking while talking, and difficulty with sequential tasks. Transition between movements is more difficult than performance of repetitive movements. The ability to programme movements is task dependent.

◇ Rigidity also increases energy expenditure and, therefore, increases the patient's perception of effort. Rigidity of muscles restricts function and can profoundly affect rotational movements. Rigidity also negatively impacts on the control of balance.

◇ While resting tremor in PD can cause minimal functional consequences, patients may also demonstrate action and intention tremors resulting in significant functional disability.

◇ Postural instability is a major problem. More than one third of all PD patients fall and over 10% fall more than once a week. The instability may be due to decreased proprioception and kinaesthetic processing. Patients are unable to adjust the magnitude of the response to the degree of perturbation and are unable to activate muscle force proportional to displacement. PD patients also demonstrate a decreased ability for strategy selection.

Perceptual, attention, and cognitive deficits

◆ Functional abilities in PD patients are also impaired by perceptual, attention, and cognitive deficits. These may include:

◇ Decreased frontal lobe function.

◇ Inability to quickly shift attention.

◇ Difficulty with visual–spatial perception and discrimination.

◇ Difficulty sequencing.

◇ Difficulty selecting the correct motor response based on the sensory input.

◇ Procedural learning deficits: individuals require significant practice and repetition to learn improved motor or cognitive functions. A multisensory approach to learning increases the success of interventions. Visual input to this approach increases effectiveness.

Referral to a therapist

◆ PTs and OTs play a major role in 'secondary care'. PD patients with various conditions are often treated initially by a physician and then referred to therapy for secondary care. This occurs in a wide range of settings, including acute care and rehabilitation hospitals, outpatient clinics, and home health.

◆ PTs and OTs also play a large role in disease prevention and the promotion of health, wellness, and fitness.

◇ Primary prevention – preventing a target condition in a susceptible population through specific measures such as general health promotion.

◇ Secondary prevention – decreasing duration of illness, severity of disease, and number of sequelae through early diagnosis and prompt intervention.

◇ Tertiary prevention – limiting the degree of disability and promoting rehabilitation and restoration of function in a patient with a chronic and irreversible disorder such as PD.

◆ In order for PD patients to receive the maximum benefit from therapy it is important that the appropriate referral is made. Patients will gain the most benefit from an early referral to initiate education and prevention strategies. This includes making a referral to the right discipline in the right rehabilitation setting (**112**).

The role of the physical and occupational therapist

112 Referral to a physical or occupational therapist. The role of the occupational therapist and physiotherapist in PD is shown. There is an overlap in some of the areas addressed by each speciality.

Occupational therapy
Handwriting
Feeding
Dressing
Bathing
Household tasks
Ergonomics (worksite modification)

Pain
Strength
Range of motion
Proprioception
Coordination

Physical therapy
Gait
Balance/falling
Transfers
Fatigue
Decreased conditioning
Flexibility

Limitations of therapy

H & Y STAGE	CORRECTION	COMPENSATION
1	✓	
2	✓	
3	✓	✓
4	✓	✓
5		✓

113 Limitations of the physical and occupational therapist. The primary aim of therapist input according to the Hoehn and Yahr stage of PD (see Chapter 6).

Limitations of therapy

◆ It is critical for the family and carers to take significant responsibility in PD therapy, especially since the disease does not affect everyone the same way. Although some people become severely disabled, others experience only minor motor disruptions.

◆ The role of the therapist is not to provide a cure, but to provide treatments or compensations to overcome physical dysfunction in an effort to reduce disability and improve quality of life. These interventions are designed to be carried out outside the clinic as well as in the home through the patient and their carers.

◆ Early in the disease process the emphasis is on correcting the dysfunctions. As the disease advances that focus begins to shift to compensations (**113**). This may include prescribing aids for walking (canes or walkers) or adaptive equipment to increase independence and safety with ADLs (see occupational therapy section).

Role of the physical therapist

◆ Postural instability and dysfunction with gait and balance are common symptoms of the disease as it progresses. These issues can have a significant impact on the mobility and quality of life for an individual with PD as well as their family.

◆ A true multidisciplinary approach to the evaluation and treatment of PD requires the involvement of a PT.

◆ The goal of physical therapy is to teach patients exercises, strategies, and compensations that maintain or increase activity levels, decrease rigidity and bradykinesia, optimize gait, and improve balance and motor coordination.

Major dysfunctions addressed by the physical therapist

◆ Difficulty with gait. Patients with PD may experience difficulty initiating and terminating gait. They may 'freeze' in doorways, thresholds, tight spaces or crowds. This inability to transport themselves safely and consistently is not only a safety risk, but can contribute to a significant decline in quality of life.

◆ Fall prevention. Approximately 38% of individuals with PD will fall each year. Approximately 18% of those falls will result in fractures.

◆ Difficulty with ADLs and transfers. Self-care management is the ability to perform ADLs such as bed mobility, transfers, dressing, grooming, bathing, eating, and toileting. Home management includes the ability to perform more complex instrumental activities of daily living (IADLs), such as maintaining a home, shopping, household chores, caring for dependents, and gardening. Difficulty here can be caused by physical impairments as well as environmental, home, and work barriers. These barriers can include safety hazards (throw rugs, slippery surfaces, poor lighting), access problems (narrow doors, thresholds, high steps, lack of power doors or elevators), or home/office design barriers (excessive distances to negotiate, multistorey environments, sinks, bathrooms, counters, placement of controls or switches). This is an area that is most effectively evaluated and managed in collaboration with an OT.

Evaluation and treatment by the physical therapist

◆ Individuals with PD are often confronted with many physical challenges as a result of their functional limitations (e.g. inability to walk), high incidence of inactivity, and associated health conditions. When combined with the natural ageing process, the likelihood of becoming physically dependent on others for assistance with daily activities substantially increases. This can be a devastating combination for those living at or close to the 'threshold' of physical dependence.

◆ Tasks that could at one time be accomplished with great ease become major obstacles. Climbing stairs, walking with a cane or walker, carrying packages, transferring from a wheelchair to a bed, commode, chair or car, and standing for long periods of time, become difficult or impossible.

◆ An examination done by a PT is required prior to any intervention. This includes a comprehensive screening as well as a specific testing process to identify impairments to be treated, or the need for referral to another practitioner (OT, speech and language therapist).

◆ Referral to a PT for early intervention should be considered when trying to manage the physical disability caused by PD in order to:
  ◇ Identify motor dysfunction as well as impairments that can be addressed through exercise and behavioural modification.
  ◇ Determine the need for treatment and benchmark future changes in patient function.
  ◇ Develop effective gait and balance strategies with greater ease before significant disease progression ensues.
  ◇ Educate patients and families/carers on expected progression and the importance of maintenance of exercise.
  ◇ Possibly slow disease progression. It has been hypothesized that early and sustained exercise in patients with PD may have a neuroprotective effect.

◆ Upon evaluation, the PT will create a personalized treatment regimen to help the patient improve/maintain functional independence and safety. Treatments should be centred on specific impairments in an effort to achieve specific goals defined by the roles patients play in their lives.

The role of the physical and occupational therapist

◆ Strength is necessary to move one's body in the environment, and to generate forces needed to transfer safely and carry objects while walking. Virtually all patients with PD will experience some degree of muscle weakness during the course of the disease. An individualized strength training programme could provide individuals with greater confidence in accomplishing more physically demanding tasks and ultimately result in greater freedom and physical independence.

◆ Range of motion and flexibility. Appropriate motion at each joint and appropriate length in each muscle are needed in order to move without limitations. Increased resistance to movement due to impaired range of motion and flexibility causes increased energy expenditure, which may lead to an increase in fatigue. These issues need to be addressed with all patients. This includes peripheral and axial motion.

◆ Posture can lead to significant difficulty performing ADLs. Postural dysfunction can also lead to impaired balance through forward or backward positioning of the patient's centre of mass.

◆ Endurance/fatigue. Many individuals with PD are deconditioned, lacking adequate physical endurance. They may tire easily increasing their risk of falls while walking, transferring, or performing basic ADLs. It may also impact on their ability to complete ADLs, household tasks, and errands safely or in reasonable time.

◆ Balance. PTs assess disturbances in balance in order to assess the risk of falling (**114**). It is important for the PT to assess the function of all systems involved in maintaining balance (vision, somatosensation, vestibular) as well as the patient's ability to use appropriate strategies to recover from losses of balance (ankle, hip, and stepping). The wobble board is one tool used to assess and treat balance (**115**).

114 Evaluation by the physical therapist. Assessment of patient's balance in the gym.

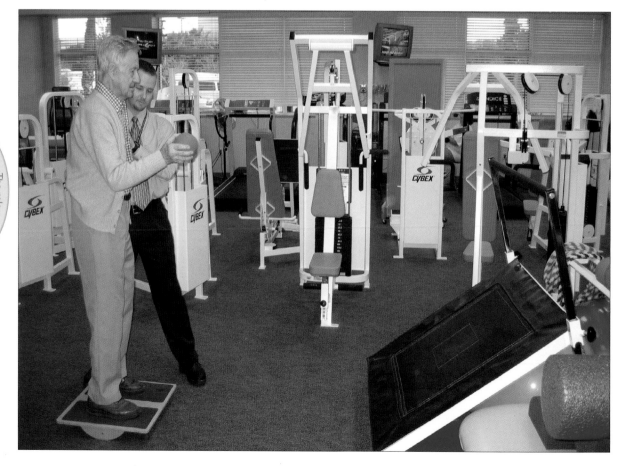

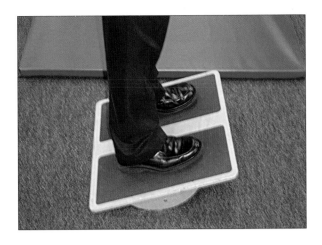

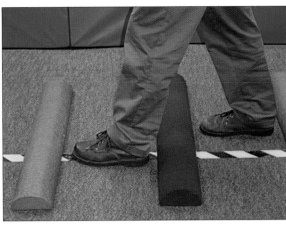

115 Assessing and treating balance problems. An exercise programme using a wobble board can assist balance and core stability for PD patients.

116 Assessing and treating gait issues. The PD patient often finds it easier to step over an object, which can assist overcoming start hesitation in walking.

◆ Gait is defined as the manner in which a person walks, characterized by rhythm, cadence (the 'beat' of movement), step, stride, and speed. Locomotion is the ability to move from one place to another. Difficulty with gait can often involve difficulty integrating sensory, motor, and neural processes. The therapist must identify strategies to help patients overcome their gait dysfunction or determine whether the patient is a candidate for assistive or adaptive devices/equipment (cane, walker, wheelchair).

◆ Common strategies employed to help patients overcome episodes of freezing and short, shuffling steps include:

◇ Visual cues (e.g. step over an object or carer's foot, inverted cane, using a laser pointer to create a dot on floor as a target).

◇ Auditory cues (e.g. metronome, counting aloud, humming a tune).

◇ Internal cues, for patients with mild disability who are able to concentrate on step by step activity rather than continuous gait. Patients can stop/pause to regroup/reset and start again with one good step (**116**).

Effects of medication on movement dysfunction

◆ Patients can experience significant differences in physical performance between 'on' and 'off' times. It is important for the therapist to be aware of these fluctuations and assist the patient in planning/coordinating their day. Helping the patient to develop strategies for both their 'on' and 'off' times is very important.

◆ Medications are not consistently effective for treating balance problems and postural instability (although they can be effective, particularly earlier in the disease course).

◆ Dyskinesias can be a side-effect of medication therapy. This complication can lead to increased difficulty with mobility and postural stability/balance.

◆ There is no significant change in strength, however, patients will appreciate improved reactions and force generation, and decreased freezing through improvements in bradykinesia and rigidity.

◆ Significant improvements with independence in ADLs can be expected with reductions in rigidity, tremor, bradykinesia, and gait.

The role of the physical and occupational therapist

Effects of surgical intervention on movement dysfunction

◆ Improvements in gait can be expected, but DBS or lesioning procedures do not improve the patient beyond their best 'on' response for gait and balance.

◆ Literature is inconclusive at present regarding consistent significant benefits of surgical treatments for addressing postural instability and balance impairments associated with PD.

◆ Reduction in bradykinesia, dyskinesia, tremor, and 'on'/'off' fluctuations will aid the patient in planning their day, and will also afford the therapist more consistency and stability while developing treatment/compensatory strategies.

Role of the occupational therapist

◆ The primary goal of the OT with a PD patient is to assist in improving the quality of life throughout the disease process:
  ◇ Improve functional movement.
  ◇ When the patient is unable to perform ADLs in a conventional manner, instruct the patient and the family in accommodation techniques that would adapt their performance or environment in order to maximize functional independence.
  ◇ Provide emotional support for the patient and the family.

◆ Early referral to an OT will address:
  ◇ Baseline evaluations of the degree of motor disorder, active functional movement, passive joint movement, dependence level in ADLs, speed of performance of self-care activities, handwriting skills, and ability to perform simultaneous and sequential tasks.
  ◇ Instruction in accommodation principles that can be used throughout the progression of the disease.
  ◇ Prevention of musculoskeletal deficits becoming impairments.
  ◇ Instruction in grading of activities so function can be facilitated despite changing symptoms.
  ◇ Early initiation of environmental adaptations.
  ◇ Carer instruction in the disease process and the process of rehabilitation.
  ◇ Patient and carer support.

Treatment of motor dysfunction

◆ Patients are treated using multisensory cueing, coupled with cognitive cueing or mental rehearsal, and reinforcement of response.

◆ Patients and carers are instructed in auditory, visual, and tactile cues to facilitate movement.

◆ Relaxation techniques can be helpful in the treatment of rigidity.

◆ Stretching is used to decrease spasm, increase proprioceptive feedback, and increase active mobility.

◆ Use of rhythm has been associated with an increase in movement ease and fluidity.

◆ Coordination drills are practised to increase accuracy of fine motor skills and the speed of these movements.

◆ Grading of simultaneous physical activities can assist with integration of performance of more than one task at a time (e.g. walking and talking).

◆ For patients with dystonia, the 'Bly multisensory treatment approach' is used. This focuses on sensory discrimination retraining for 1–2 hr, twice per week in the clinic, supervised by an OT. It also requires an intensive 2 hr/day home exercise programme practising the techniques, plus 30 minutes/day of visualization of movement.

◆ Home exercise programmes are designed to optimize strength and range of motion as well as enable the patient to continue being active in their own care.

◆ Energy conservation and work simplification techniques are taught to help manage the fatigue and decreased endurance which result from movement disorders.

Treatment of dependence in activities of daily living

◆ Progressive dependence in ADLs is one of the primary problems reported to the OT by the PD patient, the patient's family, and the carer.

◆ The dependence grows as the motor symptoms progress, as rotational movements decrease, and as flexibility declines.

◆ The speed of performance of self-care activities may also be affected. There may be difficulty performing two motor tasks at one time, delayed initiation, slow execution, and difficulty sequencing within a task, or sequencing several tasks.

- ◆ Treatment includes:
  - ◇ The development of an ADL routine that reflects the state of the mobility of the patient at the time of the task.
  - ◇ Multisensory feedback, including verbal cueing, is used to facilitate performance as the patient practises the functional movement.
  - ◇ Instruction is given regarding choosing adaptive and assistive devices (**117**).
- ◆ The primary focus is practice of the tasks. Accommodation techniques are stressed.
- ◆ The patient and the carer are also instructed regarding environmental adaptations for ADL success both in the set-up and in the use of adaptive or assistive devices. These are used when the patient is unable to perform the activity without the device, when the device significantly decreases the time required to perform the activity, and/or the device allows the patient to perform the task while in a safer position.
- ◆ Energy conservation strategies are incorporated into the individual tasks in the treatment regimen.
- ◆ All of these considerations are addressed in the following areas:

117 **Assistive devices for ADLs.** These devices help the patient in retaining independence in self-care and/or increasing safety during performance of self-care tasks. Illustrated from the top to bottom are the following – reacher, buttonhook, sock-aid, Good Grips® rocker knife, long shoehorn, Good Grips® fork, and long-handled bath sponge.

- ◇ Bed mobility. Tricks of movement are taught, and provision of a ladder strap or a bed rail may be considered.
- ◇ Mobility throughout the home. Environmental adaptations such as rearranging the furniture, removal of throw rugs, reducing clutter or other pathway distractions, and provision of even lighting may be discussed. Suggestions for remote controls to the television, or hand-held phones may be used to prevent rushing, therefore decreasing falls.
- ◇ Showering. Use of soap on a rope, terry cloth robes for drying, and shower benches may be recommended.
- ◇ Toileting. Raised toilet seats and grab bars may facilitate independence and ensure a greater level of safety in the bathroom.
- ◇ Grooming. Electric shavers may increase safety for men and women. Stabilization of the upper extremities on the edge of the sink may increase the stability of the arms for tasks at the head and neck level.
- ◇ Dressing. Adaptive methods are taught in an effort to maximize the patient's successful movement patterns. Instruction is given regarding choosing loose clothing with easy fasteners to minimize the need for fine motor control.
- ◇ Feeding. Larged-handled or security grip handled utensils may be suggested. Emphasis is on preparation of small portions, more frequent meals, and longer meal times to prevent rushing.

The role of the physical and occupational therapist

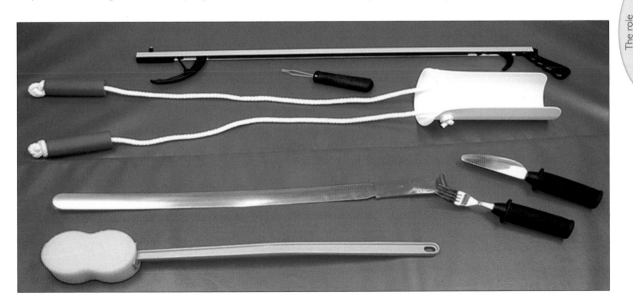

◇ Meal preparation. Adaptive jar openers, rocker knives, or dycem non-skid pads are often recommended. Sitting for aspects of meal preparation may be suggested.

◇ Household chores. Lightweight vacuum cleaners and dust mops may increase success and help to manage fatigue. Long-handled scrub brushes may facilitate independence with tasks when the patient is unable to bend or reach overhead.

◆ Handwriting is included in the ADL arena, and often is the primary reason for referral of PD patients to an OT. Difficulties can include a lack of legibility due to tremor, or problems with micrographia. Treatment of handwriting problems includes:

◇ Exercises to increase in-hand manipulation skills (**118**).

◇ Eye/hand coordination drills.

◇ Provision of proximal stability.

◇ Graded individual finger movements.

◇ Alternative methods with use of a computer.

◇ Fabrication of a writing splint (**119**).

◇ Callirobics Writing Program.

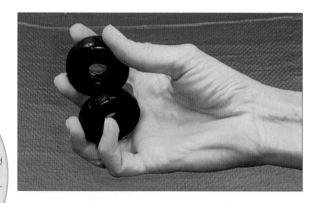

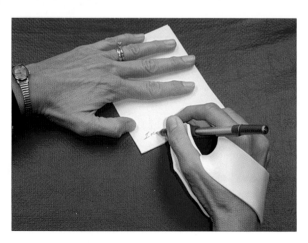

◆ While the mean age of onset of PD is around 60 years, some PD patients are diagnosed before the age of 40. Therefore, consideration of work duties must be addressed. Treatment includes:

◇ Instruction regarding work hours and schedule modification.

◇ Variance of work tasks.

◇ Ergonomic work site assessment.

Social/emotional concerns and carer support

◆ PD is known to lead to social isolation, sedentary habits, and depression.

◆ While resting tremor, a common initial PD symptom, rarely results in significant physical disability, it is frequently reported as a source of psychological distress. Most patients report being embarrassed or self-conscious regarding tremors.

◆ In the later stages of PD, tremor or rigidity may cause significant distress and add to functional disabilities. Also in the later stages, the changes in voice quality, facial expression, and lack of hand gesturing contribute to communication challenges, and thus to social participation.

◆ The OT intervenes to minimize these responses. The approach involves:

◇ Carer education and support.

◇ Involvement of the family in the rehabilitation process.

◇ Teaching the family the sensory cues to facilitate function.

◇ Encouragement of participation in local support groups.

◇ Modification of leisure activities to encourage participation and reduce isolation.

◇ Modification of communication aids (phones, computers) to facilitate communication with people outside the home.

◇ Provision of group treatment sessions that include social interaction.

◇ Instruction in the use of games or other leisure activities that can facilitate progress.

118, 119 Treatment of handwriting problems. Exercises to increase manipulation skills (above); writing splint (below).

The role of the physical and occupational therapist

CHAPTER 10

The role of the speech–language pathologist/therapist

Introduction

◆ Communication and swallowing disorders occur frequently in individuals with PD (**120**).

◆ The communication disorders seen most often in patients with PD include speech disorders and cognitive impairments.

◆ Swallowing disorders may be seen in the oral, pharyngeal, and oesophageal stages.

◆ These conditions can have a significant impact on the quality of life for an individual with PD as well as for their families. An interdisciplinary approach to diagnosis and treatment of PD requires the involvement of a speech–language pathologist/therapist.

Communication disorders in PD

◆ PD can affect the ability to communicate in several ways.

Speech disorders

◆ Hypokinetic dysarthria (**121**) occurs in well over 50% of all individuals with PD at some point in their illness.

◆ Hypokinetic dysarthria may be the presenting symptom of neurological disease in PD.

◆ Hypokinetic dysarthria is characterized by a breathy and hoarse voice, reduced loudness, monoloudness, monopitch, consonant imprecision, and rate abnormalities.

◆ The term hypophonia is often used to describe the decreased vocal loudness of individuals with PD.

121 Hypokinetic dysarthria. The perceptual features, presumed pathophysiology, and complicating features of dysarthria in Parkinson's disease.

Speech	Swallowing
Most common communication disorder is hypokinetic dysarthria	Dysphagia in all three stages of swallowing: oral; pharyngeal; oesophageal

COMMUNICATION AND SWALLOWING DISORDERS IN PD

Cognitive	Other problems
Primarily includes memory problems and/or executive function dysfunction	Other communication disorders may include masked facies, language deficits, and micrographia

120 Communication and swallowing disorders. The main concerns of the speech–language pathologist/therapist.

HYPOKINETIC DYSARTHRIA
More than 50% of PD patients have dysarthria; may be the presenting symptom

Perceptual features
Breathy/hoarse voice; decreased loudness; monoloudness; monopitch; consonant imprecision; rate abnormalities

Etiology
Basal ganglia pathophysiology; effect of motor symptoms (rigidity, bradykinesia, tremor) on the speech mechanism

Complicating factors
Cognitive disorders; perceptual deficits; neurogenic dysfluency; masked facies

- Individuals with PD often appear to have a perceptual disconnection between their actual loudness level and their own internal perception of loudness.
- Inappropriate silences may occur frequently and be associated with difficulty initiating movements for speech production.
- Neurogenic dysfluency, consisting most often of sound and word repetitions, may also be observed in some patients with PD.
- Patients most often describe the presence of a 'weak' voice. Communication partners may have a hard time hearing their speech, especially at a distance, in a noisy environment, or on the telephone. Patients may also report avoiding social situations that require speech.
- The severity of speech disorders may not correspond to the duration of PD or severity of other motor symptoms.
- Hyperkinetic dysarthria, characterized by variability in rate and loudness, may also be encountered. This most often occurs in the presence of dyskinesias, particularly after prolonged levodopa therapy.

Cognitive disorders

- As PD progresses, cognitive impairments are common.
- Many PD patients are eventually diagnosed with dementia. Some develop Alzheimer's type dementia with substantial memory problems. Others may develop Parkinson's type dementia with executive function dysfunction, as well as substantial memory problems.
- Frontal and memory dysfunction are the predominant cognitive disorders associated with PD.

Other communication disorders

- A masked facial expression (masked facies) is common. This feature, combined with hypophonia, may impair the patient's communication of their emotional state.
- Subtle language deficits may occur in patients with PD including decreased naming skills and decreased use of complex syntactic structures in spontaneous speech. Assessment of language disorders may be challenging due to co-existing speech and cognitive disturbances.
- Micrographia, or small handwriting, may be exhibited (see page 29).

Speech subsystems and their contribution to the speech signal	
SUBSYSTEM	CONTRIBUTION
Respiratory mechanism	Loudness
Larynx	Voice quality
Velopharynx	Resonance
Orofacial mechanism	Articulation

122 Speech subsystems. A distributed network of body structures with different contributions is required for speech production.

Causes of communication disorders

- The etiology of the communication disorders in PD is probably multifactorial. They appear to be related to changes in the interaction between the basal ganglia, higher cortical areas, corticospinal and corticobulbar motor tracts, the sensorimotor trigeminal system, and other areas.
- The speech deficits of hypokinetic dysarthria are presumably due to the basal ganglia pathology of PD and the influence of the primary motor symptoms of rigidity, tremor, and bradykinesia on the subsystems of speech (**122**). In addition, deficits in speech-specific programming and planning may also contribute to the speech abnormalities of patients with PD.
- Cognitive deficits seen in individuals with PD may be due to cortical involvement or more extensive subcortical damage.
- Masked facies and micrographia appear to be further manifestations of the primary motor symptoms of PD including rigidity and bradykinesia.

Evaluation and treatment of communication disorders

◆ Referral to a speech and language therapist for early intervention with communication impairments, particularly dysarthria, should be considered for a variety of reasons:
  ◇ Effective speaking strategies may be learned with greater ease before the severity of dysarthria increases.
  ◇ Early participation in speech therapy may foster later successful intervention.
  ◇ Even a mild dysarthria can have a significant functional impact on an individual's communication abilities.
  ◇ Completion of a comprehensive speech–language evaluation (**123**) is needed not only to determine the need for treatment, but to benchmark future changes in function in this progressive disorder.
  ◇ Education regarding the expected course of communication involvement and the role of speech and language therapy can be provided for patients and their families.

Behavioural interventions (124)

◆ The Lee Silverman Voice Treatment (LSVT) has substantial literature supporting its beneficial effects and is a popular treatment choice for individuals with PD and hypokinetic dysarthria.
  ◇ LSVT emphasizes phonatory effort and uses maximum performance tasks as the basis of intervention.
  ◇ LSVT also 'recalibrates' an individual's perceived level of effort with an emphasis on self-awareness.
  ◇ LSVT is based upon the premise that treatment should be simple and intensive.
  ◇ Although intact cognition is a positive prognostic indicator of success, LSVT can also be beneficial for patients with cognitive deficits.
◆ Other treatments which may be appropriate include rate control techniques and the use of delayed auditory feedback.
◆ Augmentative-alternative communication (AAC) treatment approaches may also be beneficial, particularly as dysarthria progresses.
  ◇ Voice amplifiers may be beneficial for increasing vocal loudness.
  ◇ Pacing boards may assist in rate control.

Tasks for speech examination

| Spontaneous speech |
| Reading aloud |
| Word and sentence imitation |
| Syllable repetition (i.e., diadochokinesis) |
| Vowel prolongation (i.e., maximum phonation duration) |
| Oral motor examination |
| Cranial nerve testing |

123 Speech examination. A variety of tasks are used to assess speech function in patients with Parkinson's disease.

Selected behavioural treatments for hypokinetic dysarthria

| Lee Silverman Voice Treatment (LSVT) |
| Maximum performance training |
| Expiratory muscle strength training (EMST) |
| Rate manipulations – delayed auditory feedback, pitch-shifted feedback, pacing boards |

124 Behavioural treatments. A variety of treatments are available for speech rehabilitation in Parkinson's disease.

  ◇ Alphabet boards may be an effective strategy to supplement speech and provide context for communication partners.
  ◇ Other AAC strategies such as communication boards/notebooks, voice output computer systems, and portable typing devices may also be used.

Effect of medications on communication

◆ For most individuals with PD, pharmacological treatment does not appear to have a significant beneficial impact on speech production.
◆ Hyperkinetic dysarthria, often in the presence of dyskinesias after prolonged levodopa therapy, may also be encountered.

The role of the speech–language pathologist/therapist

Surgical treatments and communication

◆ Surgical treatments for PD do not appear to have consistent significant benefit for the communication impairments associated with the disease.
  ◇ Unilateral pallidotomy is usually not found to improve speech function and can cause cognitive and behavioural changes.
  ◇ Bilateral pallidotomy is associated with an increase in the severity of pre-existing speech problems and a higher incidence of dysarthria and hypophonia.
  ◇ Thalamotomy, especially when completed bilaterally, may cause dysarthria or increase its severity.
  ◇ Deep brain stimulation (DBS) applied to the globus pallidus interna may have a range of effects on speech function. These effects are variable, and responses could range from having improvement in speech function, to having no effect, to having a negative impact.
  ◇ The effect of DBS on the subthalamic nucleus (STN) appears to be variable. There is some indication that speech may be differentially affected by left versus right stimulation, with selective left-sided-only stimulation interfering with speech production. In contrast, bilateral STN stimulation may have some limited beneficial impact on speech.

Swallowing disorders in PD

◆ Swallowing problems (dysphagia) in PD commonly involve the mechanisms controlling the tongue, pharynx and upper oesophageal sphincter (**125**).
◆ Oropharyngeal dysphagia is reported in up to 95% of patients with PD, depending on the method of assessment. However, dysphagia is often unrecognized or underestimated by patients.
◆ The severity of dysphagia may not correspond to the duration of PD or severity of other motor symptoms.
◆ All stages of swallowing function can be affected in patients with PD including the oral, pharyngeal, and oesophageal stages (**126**).

125 Oropharyngeal swallow mechanism. Critical structures of the oropharynx and cervical oesophagus involved in swallowing.

  ◇ Oral-stage deficits may include drooling, increased oral transit time, repetitive tongue pumping motions with the posterior tongue remaining elevated, and premature spillage of the bolus.
  ◇ Pharyngeal-stage problems include pharyngeal swallow delay, the presence of pharyngeal residue after the swallow, laryngeal penetration, and aspiration.
  ◇ Oesophageal-stage swallowing problems are also common, and most frequently include abnormalities in oesophageal motility.
◆ Although dysphagia is common in PD, it rarely is severe enough to require an alternative means of nutritional support. However, gastrostomy may be considered for some patients as an efficient means of providinge additional nutritional support. In some situations, oral intake may continue with the presence of a gastrostomy tube.

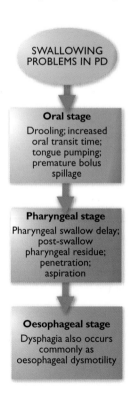

126 Dysphagia in PD. Swallowing disorders are encountered in all stages of the swallow.

The role of the speech–language pathologist/therapist

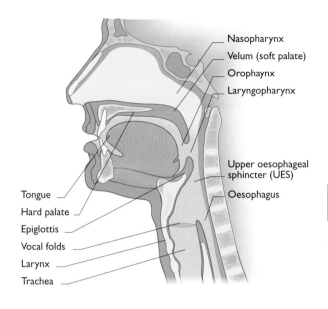

Nasopharynx
Velum (soft palate)
Orophaynx
Laryngopharynx

Upper oesophageal sphincter (UES)
Oesophagus

Tongue
Hard palate
Epiglottis
Vocal folds
Larynx
Trachea

Causes of dysphagia in PD

◆ The etiology of dysphagia in PD is complex. It appears to be related to changes in the interaction between the basal ganglia, higher cortical regions, corticospinal and corticobulbar motor tracts, the sensorimotor trigeminal system, the dorsal vagal nucleus, the reticular formation, and other areas.

◇ Oral- and pharyngeal-stage dysphagia are likely to be due to basal ganglia dysfunction and resultant motor symptoms of rigidity, tremor, and bradykinesia.

◇ Basal ganglia pathology may further influence the trigeminal system, causing sensory changes that may contribute to oropharyngeal dysphagia.

◇ Involvement of the dorsal motor nucleus of the vagus and the reticular formation may also contribute to pharyngeal-stage swallowing problems.

◇ Oesophageal stage dysphagia appears to be related to involvement of the dorsal vagal nucleus and the oesophageal myenteric plexus.

Evaluation and treatment of swallowing problems

◆ Referral to a speech and language therapist for evaluation of swallow function may be appropriate. Clinical, radiographic, and endoscopic swallow examinations may be beneficial for individuals with PD.

◆ A clinical swallow examination should include a thorough patient interview so the history and duration of the problem can be ascertained. The effect of medications taken for PD on swallowing function should also be explored, with particular attention to 'on'/'off' effects and changes in swallowing function.

◆ A radiographic swallow examination (i.e. videofluoroscopy) is often indicated for patients with PD, especially since dysphagia is often unrecognized or underestimated by patients. Videofluoroscopy allows for comprehensive evaluation of the biomechanical aspects of the oral and pharyngeal phases of swallowing, as well as the effect of compensatory techniques and postures. This exam allows for lateral and anterior-posterior views of the swallow (**127**).

127 Videofluoroscopy. Lateral radiographic images showing (a) key pharyngeal and laryngeal structures involved in swallowing and (b) aspiration, or entry of material below the vocal folds (arrow). Contrast can be viewed in the trachea.
Reprinted with permission from Plural Publishing, from Rosenbek & Jones, 2007, 'Dysphagia in patients with motor speech disorders', Motor Speech Disorders, G. Weismer (Ed.).

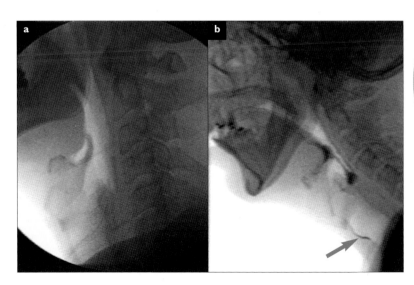

The role of the speech–language pathologist/therapist

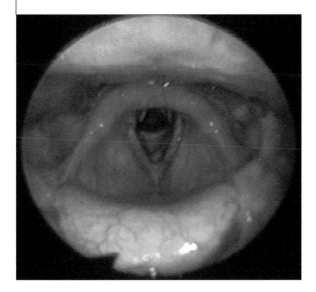

128 Endoscopic swallow examination. Aspiration as viewed during the endoscopic swallow exam. Contrast can be seen just below the level of the vocal folds.
Reprinted with permission from Plural Publishing, from Rosenbek & Jones, 2007, 'Dysphagia in patients with motor speech disorders', Motor Speech Disorders, G. Weismer (Ed.).

Effect of medications on swallowing

◆ If dopaminergic medications improve swallowing function for individual patients, 'on' effects should be timed to coincide with meals and swallowing evaluations.

◆ Pharyngeal residue and oesophageal dysmotility may cause irregular absorption of orally ingested medications.

◆ Anticholinergics have been found to be less effective when delivered parenterally instead of orally.

Surgical treatments and swallowing

◆ Surgical treatment of PD may also be associated with dysphagia.
   ◇ Thalamotomy, particularly when completed bilaterally, may cause dysphagia.
   ◇ Bilateral pallidotomy is also associated with increased incidence of dysphagia.
   ◇ The effect of DBS on swallow function requires further research.

◆ An endoscopic swallow examination (also known as the fiberoptic endoscopic evaluation of swallowing or FEES®) is another instrumental approach to the assessment of swallowing which may be utilized in some patients with PD. The endoscopic exam allows a superior view of the pharynx and larynx via the transnasal passage of a flexible endoscope (**128**).

◆ A baseline weight may serve as an index of future weight loss related to dysphagia.

Behavioural interventions

◆ LSVT, commonly used as an effective treatment for the speech disorders of individuals with PD, may also be a beneficial treatment for swallowing problems.

◆ The videofluoroscopic and endoscopic exams allow for the effect of compensatory techniques and rehabilitation techniques to be evaluated, which can then be implemented in a dysphagia treatment programme.

◆ Smaller, more frequent meals may be valuable to optimize nutritional intake and optimize swallowing function, especially if swallowing requires a lot of effort or causes fatigue.

◆ Referrals to occupational therapy may also be beneficial to determine whether adaptive utensils and equipment will promote independence with meals due to the effect of motor symptoms (i.e. tremor) on self-feeding skills.

CHAPTER 11

Malnutrition and related disorders

Nutritional health and the role of the registered dietician

◆ There are many obstacles and frank barriers to nutritional health among people with PD. These can be due to the nature of the disease, to disabilities resulting from the disease, or to the medications needed to treat it.

◆ Nutrient depletion can weaken the immune system, lead to depression, unplanned weight loss, cognitive impairment, protein-energy malnutrition, bone fractures, dehydration, pressure ulcers, and other serious conditions, often requiring hospitalization (**129**).

◆ These can seriously impact on the health and quality of life of the individual.

◆ Medical nutrition therapy, provided by a registered dietician, is therefore an important component of a team approach to treatment. It can help prevent malnutrition, provide a better quality of life, and reduce hospitalizations and health-related expenditures. Where possible, a registered dietician should be included shortly after diagnosis of PD.

Nutritional disorders related to autonomic effects of PD

◆ PD may affect the autonomic nervous system, resulting in slowed motility of the GI tract. This can impact on one or more areas of the GI tract, resulting in many barriers to nutrient repletion (**130**).

129 Malnutrition. Potential effects of poor nutrition which can affect PD patients.

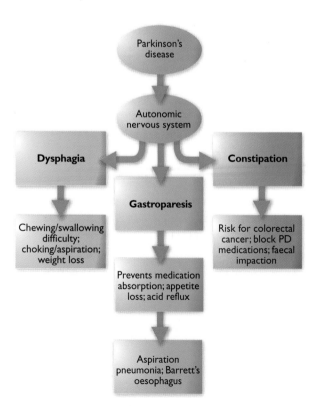

130 Autonomic effects. Involvement of the autonomic nervous system in reducing nutrient intake in PD patients.

Dysphagia

◆ Chewing and swallowing difficulties.

◆ Choking, and/or aspiration of foods, liquids, refluxed stomach contents, and saliva.

◆ Unfavourably impacts on energy and nutrient intake:

◇ Unplanned weight loss.

◇ Malnutrition.

◇ Aspiration pneumonia.

◆ *Management.* Referral to a speech and language therapist for a swallowing evaluation and modified food consistency if needed. If the speech and language therapist determines thickened liquids or pureed foods are needed, the individual should be referred to a registered dietician for nutrition assessment and appropriate diet planning.

Gastroparesis

◆ Delays the passage of food into the small intestine.

◆ May prevent or slow the absorption of medication.

◆ Causes early satiety, loss of appetite, inability to finish meals.

◆ Can cause gastro-oesophageal reflux disease:

◇ May lead to injury of oesophagus and lower oesophageal sphincter.

◇ Can cause Barrett's oesophagus, a precancerous condition.

◇ If dysphagia is present, there is increased risk for aspiration of refluxed stomach contents, and aspiration pneumonia.

◇ Medications used to treat gastro-oesophageal reflux disease by raising gastric pH can interfere with the metabolism of some nutrients, including vitamin B12 and iron.

◆ *Management.* Numerous small meals and snacks, nutrient-dense and moderate in fat and fibre, are preferred. Protein needs should be assessed, and should be divided equally among small morning, midday, and evening meals, levodopa taken about 30 minutes before these. Low-protein snacks should be taken between these meals to meet total calorie needs. Use of 'liquid Sinemet' or Parcopa (USA) or Madopar Dispersible (Europe) may be helpful when stomach emptying is slowed.

◇ If gastro-oesophageal reflux disease is present, use of small meals and avoidance of 'trigger foods,' i.e. caffeine, citrus, tomatoes, alcohol, should be helpful. The day's final meal should be consumed at least 4 hr before bedtime, so that the stomach is empty before lying down.

Constipation

◆ May predate diagnosis of PD by as much as several years; may even be an early symptom of PD.

◆ Elevates risk for colorectal cancer.

◆ Can block effectiveness of PD medications.

◆ Chronic laxative use, including senna and cascara sagrada, may damage the colon.

◆ Dysregularion of autonomic nervous system may cause pelvic floor dysfunction, with inability to evacuate the stool.

◆ Chronic or prolonged constipation may cause faecal impaction.

◆ *Management.* Discuss with patient the signs of faecal impaction and availability of screening for colorectal cancer. Physical activity, as ability permits, is desirable. Dietary sources of insoluble fibre, a minimum of 25 g daily, along with six to eight 250 ml glasses of fluids, will help to increase stool bulk and speed colon transit time. Use of both prebiotics and probiotics may be helpful, along with servings of laxative foods such as prunes and kiwifruit. The dietician should assess fibre and fluid intake and provide individualized advice as needed.

◇ If dietary measures fail to produce bowel movement, the possibility of pelvic floor dysfunction should be considered, and medical management may be needed. However, diet and lifestyle changes should be the preferred method of managing constipation for as long as possible, in order to avoid chronic laxative use.

Nutritional disorders related to mental aspects of PD

Parkinson's disease may also affect mental and emotional health and energy level; this can have an impact on nutrient repletion (**131**).

Cognitive impairment
◆ Cognitive impairment is estimated to affect about 19% of patients.
◆ Another 27% may suffer from dementia.
◆ All degrees of cognitive impairment can affect eating habits.
◆ Mild forgetfulness can affect:
  ◇ Ability to drive.
  ◇ Shopping for food.
  ◇ Preparation of food.
  ◇ Taking medications on time.
  ◇ Symptoms thus are not well managed, and decreased control of symptoms may affect manual dexterity and other physical abilities.

◆ Dementia may:
  ◇ Influence the desire to eat.
  ◇ Require increasing assistance from carer.
◆ Malnutrition itself may be a causative or contributing factor to cognitive impairment and dementia.
  ◇ Older adults are less likely to produce the stomach acid and intrinsic factor needed to metabolize vitamin B12. Changes in sensory functions and/or appetite may alter the kind or amount of foods eaten, resulting in nutrient deficiencies.
  ◇ B vitamin deficiencies may produce confusion, cognitive impairment, behaviour change, even an Alzheimer-type dementia.
  ◇ B12 deficiency may result in macrocytic megaloblastic anaemia; paresthesias, peripheral neuropathy; psychiatric disorders, including impaired memory, irritability, depression, and dementia.

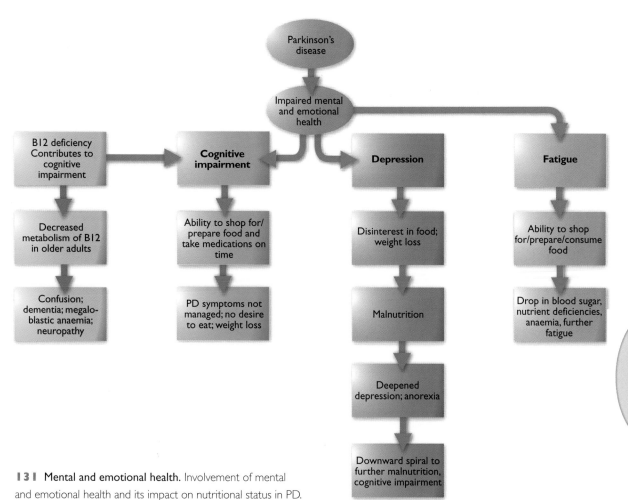

131 **Mental and emotional health.** Involvement of mental and emotional health and its impact on nutritional status in PD.

Malnutrition and related disorders

◆ *Management.* Assess status of B1 (thiamine), B2 (riboflavin), B3 (niacin), B6 (pyridoxine), B12, and folate, all of which are implicated in cognitive impairment, memory loss, confusion, and dementias. Assess dietary intake, and provide advice where needed. Consider use of fortified foods or vitamin/mineral supplements. The carer will be of primary importance in helping to guard against malnutrition, and careful instruction and education of the carer are required.

Depression

◆ Affects about 40% of patients.
◆ May be endogenous or exogenous.
◆ May range from sadness to major depression.
◆ May predate diagnosis of PD by several years.
◆ Depression can impact on nutritional health:
  ◇ Significantly affects functional ability.
  ◇ May adversely affect the appetite and desire to eat.
  ◇ Results in narrowed range of food choices, diminished food intake, unplanned weight loss.
  ◇ Ensuing nutritional deficiencies can exacerbate existing depression, anorexia, and unwillingness to eat.
  ◇ Creates a downward spiral to malnutrition.
◆ Anxiety or panic attacks may accompany, or be independent of, depression.
◆ *Management.* It will be important to determine both the form and degree of depression, and whether it will be best treated by therapeutic counselling, dietary measures, or medication. Addition of antidepressants, particularly in older adults, and more particularly those already using two or more medications, may produce adverse side-effects.
  ◇ Consider referral to a registered dietician for assessment of dietary intake, particularly if unplanned weight change has occurred. If diet is inadequate, fortified foods or a multivitamin/mineral supplement may be helpful. Additionally, provision of omega-3 fatty acids, via fish oil capsules, may be helpful.
  ◇ Also consider referral to a qualified therapist who can provide counselling and prescribe an antidepressant if needed.

◇ If anxiety or panic attacks are reported, determine whether these occur regularly, particularly if before meals, or at the same time of day. If so, hypoglycemia should be ruled out as a causative factor.

Fatigue

◆ Complaints of exhaustion and sleepiness are common among patients. This may alter the ability to shop for, prepare, and eat food.
◆ Can be an effect of PD.
◆ May be a side-effect of medications, with additive effects from multiple medications.
◆ May be dietary causes:
  ◇ Decreased food intake can result in drop in blood glucose, with attendant fatigue.
  ◇ Prolonged reduction in caloric intake may result in deficiencies of B vitamins and iron, and fatigue.
  ◇ The various anaemias can result in fatigue, shortness of breath, dizziness, confusion.
◆ *Management.* Rule out dietary causes. Reports of recent weight loss along with fatigue are an indication of nutrition-related etiology.
  ◇ Determine if energy intake is adequate (particularly if unplanned weight loss has occurred).
  ◇ Rule out deficiencies of folate, B6, B12, iron.
  ◇ Rule out hypoglycemia.
  ◇ Test for anaemia (iron-deficiency, macrocytic megaloblastic).
  ◇ If insomnia is present, discuss avoidance of caffeine and alcohol after late afternoon; regular practice of meditation, or yoga; a light snack before bedtime, such as a cracker with a teaspoonful of peanut butter, or half a banana. A calcium–magnesium supplement at bedtime may help with relaxation: 100–200 mg calcium, 50 mg magnesium.

Other effects of PD on nutritional health

◆ PD affects physical abilities and sensory functions, which can indirectly impact on nutritional health (**132**).

Physical impairment

◆ Symptoms include tremor, dyskinesia, rigidity, bradykinesia, decreased manual dexterity.
◆ These affect the ability to manipulate eating utensils.
◆ The patient may require hours to finish a meal.
◆ The patient cannot ingest sufficient food to maintain weight or nutrient repletion.
◆ *Management*. Determine whether patient is taking medications on time; if forgetful, may be undermedicated. Thus, PD symptoms will not be well controlled, and swallowing may be more difficult.
  ◇ Consider a referral to an OT, who may provide special eating utensils.
  ◇ Consider a referral to a registered dietician, for help choosing foods that can be eaten out of the hand, or that require less chewing.

Impaired gait and balance

◆ Impaired gait and balance lead to a decrease in weight-bearing exercise.
◆ This results in muscle wasting and bone thinning.
◆ There is an increased likelihood of falls and increased likelihood of subsequent fractures.
◆ If diet is lacking in protein and nutrients, the probability of muscle wasting and bone thinning is further increased.
◆ *Management*. Encourage as much physical activity as ability permits. Consider referral to a physical therapist for help with appropriate exercises.
  ◇ Consider a referral to a registered dietician to determine adequacy of calcium, magnesium, vitamins D and K, for bone health; assessment of protein needs for muscle maintenance.
  ◇ If bone density baseline has not been established, order fall risk assessment and fracture risk assessment, including dual energy X-ray absorptiometry (DEXAscan), to determine baseline bone density.

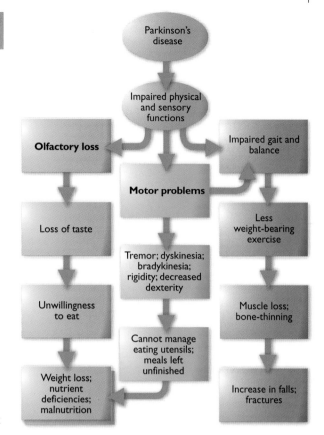

132 Physical and sensory functions. The physical symptoms of PD and their impact on nutritional status.

  ◇ Advise patient and family regarding use of hip protectors, to help prevent fractures in case of falls (see Resources section).

Loss of olfaction

◆ This is common among PD patients.
◆ It is usually accompanied by loss of the sense of taste.
◆ In combination with other factors such as depression or medication-induced appetite loss, it can produce unwillingness to eat.
◆ This can seriously affect energy and nutrient intake.
◆ *Management*. Consider referral to a registered dietician who can help patient and family select preferred foods. Numerous small meals or nourishing snacks may be better than three large meals daily.

Malnutrition and related disorders

Effects of PD medication

◆ The nutritional concerns related to effects of PD medications are summarized in **133**.

Nausea/vomiting

◆ May need to take medications with meals until nausea has diminished, usually a few weeks. At that time, levodopa should be taken 30–60 minutes prior to meals.

◆ Many people find use of ginger tea, or chewing crystallized ginger, helps to manage nausea.

◆ Some cases may require medication, such as carbidopa (Lodosyn, available in the USA) or domperidone (available in Europe), to combat nausea/vomiting. Avoid use of prochlorperazine or metoclopramide; these may exacerbate PD symptoms and are contraindicated for those with PD.

Protein–levodopa interaction

◆ Both from the gut, and at the blood–brain barrier, levodopa competes for absorption with the large neutral amino acids, which are breakdown products of ingested proteins.

◆ Patients using quick-release formulations, such as Sinemet or Madopar (or their generic forms) should take these about 30 minutes prior to meals.

◆ The CR formulation may be taken with meals; however, more time is required before it takes effect. Thus, if motor fluctuations or gastroparesis are of concern, or if the individual is particularly protein-sensitive, it is best to take the CR form well ahead of meals also.

◆ If motor fluctuations are not controlled by taking levodopa prior to meals, further adjustment may be necessary.

133 Medication side-effects. Various aspects of medication can have an impact on the nutritional status of PD patients.

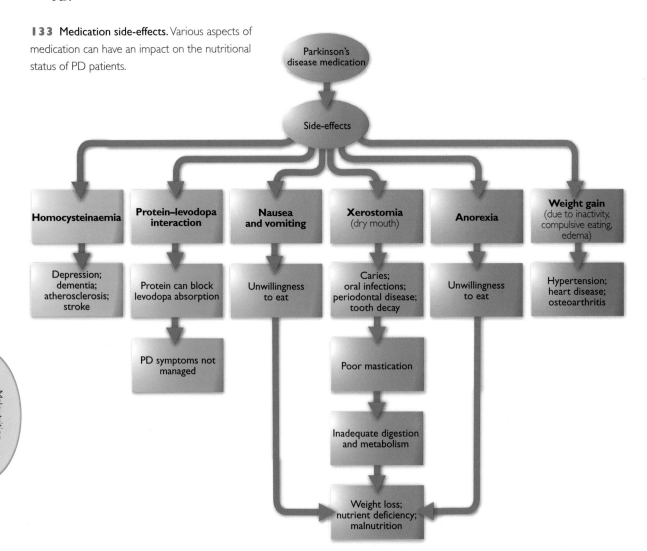

Malnutrition and related disorders

◆ Originally, patients experiencing fluctuations were advised to avoid protein during the day, when mobility was most important. The entire day's protein was then ingested at the evening meal. Protein was restricted to between 0.5 and 0.8 g/kg body weight. However, this unnatural eating plan can contribute to unwillingness to eat, followed by unplanned weight loss and malnutrition. Additionally, PD symptoms will not be controlled during the night and the patient therefore is unable to turn in bed, or use the bathroom, leading to protein avoidance at the evening meal as well. The result is protein-energy malnutrition.

◆ Of further concern, it is now known that older adults and people suffering from disorders such as PD have increased protein requirements.

◆ *Management.* A safe, simple, and effective method of management is for a dietician to assess the patient's calorie and protein needs, allotting 1.0–1.2 g protein/kg body weight.

◇ Conditions such as unplanned weight loss, osteopenia/osteoporosis, sarcopenia, pressure ulcers, and fever, may increase protein needs.

◇ The day's protein should be divided evenly among the morning, midday, and evening meals. Levodopa can then be taken 30 minutes before each meal, and between meals if necessary, without protein interaction.

Unplanned weight gain

◆ This can be due to:

◇ Inactivity, brought on by decreased physical ability.

◇ Edema.

◇ PD medications, in particular the agonists, may result in weight gain. In some individuals, this is due to edema (fluid retention), which may dissipate over time. Persistence of marked edema and weight gain may lead to hypertension and other weight-related disorders.

◇ Compulsive eating. PD medications, often the agonists, may lead to OCDs, and in some this results in overeating.

◆ *Management.* Encourage as much physical activity as ability permits.

◇ Regarding edema, a natural diuretic eating plan referred to as the DASH diet (dietary approach to stop hypertension) was developed to combat both edema and hypertension and studies have suggested benefit. The DASH diet can be adapted by the registered dietician for individual use. Resources are available on the Internet and can be downloaded at no charge (see Dietician Resources, page 161).

◇ If weight gain is due to compulsive overeating, the individual may benefit from counselling by a therapist, as well as referral to a dietician. Sometimes DA therapy will need to be discontinued.

◇ Whether the weight gain is due to edema or overeating, the patient should be carefully monitored. Some individuals respond favourably to a change in medication.

Unplanned weight loss

◆ The etiology of unplanned weight loss can include:

◇ Medication side-effects, particularly in the older adult: nausea, anorexia, taste changes, depression.

◇ Dysphagia: difficulty chewing, swallowing.

◇ Gastroparesis, early satiety.

◇ Cognitive impairment.

◇ Decreased manual dexterity.

◆ *Management.* See previous sections for managing the above causes. Consider referral to a registered dietician for help with appropriate assessment and medical nutrition therapy.

Xerostomia

◆ Xerostomia (dry mouth) is of concern because it may lead to candidiasis, periodontal disease, caries, and other oral diseases; oral diseases may interfere with mastication.

◆ It may result from:

◇ Side-effect of medications.

◇ Mouth breathing.

◇ Rarely, Sjögren's syndrome.

Malnutrition and related disorders

◆ *Management.* Xerostomia may be difficult to address. Patients often have difficulty with brushing and flossing. Also, may have limited success with dentures. Tremor, dystonia, and/or dyskinesia may interfere with dental care.

◇ Inquire about dry mouth and oral health, educate regarding need for fluids, and recommend consultation with a dentist in order to prevent tooth loss and oral disease.

Homocysteinaemia

◆ Elevated plasma homocysteine may occur with long-term use of levodopa.

◆ Homocysteinaemia is associated with depression, dementia, atherosclerosis, stroke.

◆ Serum homocysteine requires the combined action of vitamins B6, B12, and folate for clearance from the bloodstream. Elevation can occur with deficiency of one or more of these.

◆ Most PD patients are older adults; many elderly people produce less intrinsic factor, needed for absorption of B12 in the ileum, which may result in pernicious anaemia.

◆ Many elderly suffer from atrophic gastritis: the stomach secretes less of the acid needed to cleave B12 from food proteins, resulting in megalo-blastic anaemia.

◆ Changed eating habits may, over time, result in B-vitamin deficiencies, the signs of which closely resemble, and may exacerbate, symptoms of PD: paresthesia, impaired gait, personality or behaviour changes, sore or burning mouth or tongue, burning feet, dementia, and depression.

◆ An excess of folate may mask B12, thus B12 status must be measured independently, testing for methylmalonic acid.

◆ Because of the prevalence of cognitive impair-ment and dementia in PD, serum homocysteine should be assessed, along with B6, B12, and folate status, and tests for megaloblastic and per-nicious anaemias.

◆ A registered dietician should periodically request a 3-day food–medication diary, to determine whether the diet is adequate; if inadequate, the physician should be notified and laboratory testing ordered. A B-complex supplement or intramuscular injection may be needed to restore levels to normal.

CHAPTER 12

Complementary medicine and Parkinson's disease

Introduction

◆ The use of complementary therapies by PD patients is very common. Rajendran *et al.* (2001) found that 40% of PD patients surveyed used complementary therapies including vitamins, herbs, massage, and acupuncture. Little scientific evidence exists regarding the safety and efficacy of most of these alternative treatments for PD.

◆ A conservative estimate is that, in 1997, out-of-pocket expenditures for complementary medicine for PD patients in the USA was $27 billion.

◆ The use of herbal remedies and nutritional supplements is governed in the USA by the 1994 Dietary Supplement and Health Education Act. This act exempts the companies manufacturing these products from having to provide detailed safety and efficacy information. In Europe, most vitamins, minerals and supplements are treated as foods and medicinal claims are not permitted. Nutrient contents are declared according to the European Union Recommended Daily Allowances.

◆ The National Center for Complementary and Alternative Medicine in the USA is currently funding several studies of common herbal medications to examine drug interactions. For example, Hu *et al.* (2005) reported that the use of *Piper methysticum* (kava) increased 'off' periods in patients with parkinsonism taking levodopa. In the UK, the Foundation for Integrated Health argues for combining complemetary and alternative approaches with mainstream medicine.

Acupuncture

◆ Acupuncture has been practised for over 2,000 years.

◆ It is based on the concept that health is dependent on the smooth flow of energy – 'qi' (pronounced 'chi') – through the body, along channels known as meridians (**134**). This energy can be blocked or disturbed by physical, mental, or emotional factors.

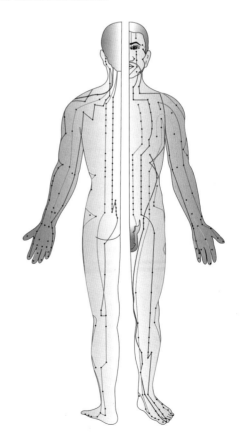

134 Acupuncture theory. Illustration of the twelve primary acupuncture meridians and the acupuncture points along them.

135 Acupuncture therapy. A practitioner inserts a needle into the 43rd point on the 'stomach' meridian.

- Acupuncture strives to balance yin and yang (two 'opposing forces' in ancient Chinese philosophy) and the five elements (water, wood, fire, earth, and metal) within the body.
- Regulation of imbalance or obstruction is through the insertion of fine needles just below the skin which are believed to stimulate the body's own healing mechanisms (**135**).
- The biological mechanism of the action is poorly defined.
- PD patient reports include temporary benefits such as decreased tremor and stiffness.
- Adverse events are rare but may include the risk of hepatitis B virus transmission, perichondritis, bacterial endocarditis, spinal infection, osteomyelitis, compartment syndrome, cardiac tamponade, pneumothorax, and, notably, spinal cord and root injuries.
- Most reported studies of acupuncture are open label (nonblinded) and investigators have suggested that it is difficult to include a sham treatment group to serve as a control. In studies of acupuncture in other diseases, the sham group frequently exhibited as much improvement as the treatment group.

- One nonblinded, pilot trial of acupuncture in PD has been published. This study examined the safety and efficacy of acupuncture in 20 patients with PD. Eighty-five percent of the patients reported subjective improvement of symptoms. Qualitative measures did not show significant improvement except in the areas of sleep and rest. No significant serious adverse events were reported.
- To date, there is insufficient scientific evidence to routinely recommend the use of acupuncture to treat PD.
- Acupuncture is usually not covered by insurance and requires multiple treatments.

Massage therapy

- Massage therapy involves manipulation of muscles and other soft tissues of the body. Varieties of massage range from gentle stroking and kneading of muscles and other soft tissue to manual 'deep tissue' techniques.
- Types of massage include aromatherapy, craniofacial, lymphatic, myofascial, reflexology (which involves 'reflex areas' mainly in the feet, occasionally the hands), rolfing (a technique of loosening and balancing connective tissues introduced by Dr Ida Loft), shiatsu (a Japanese healing art based on finger pressure), sports, Swedish (a technique that copies the moves of gymnasts), and trigger point.
- Patient reports indicate that massage may provide benefit with regard to muscle stiffness and aching.
- There is no scientific evidence to support benefits of routine massage therapy for PD.
- Massage therapy is usually not covered by insurance and requires multiple treatments.

Tai chi

- Tai chi chuan (literally, 'supreme ultimate fist') is an ancient Chinese 'soft' martial art. It is now practised worldwide, in various styles.
- The main practice of tai chi is to learn a series of forms or postures which emphasize a straight spine, controlled abdominal breathing, and a natural, fluid range of motion (**136**).
- The focusing of the practitioner on the movement and form is thought of as a 'moving meditation' that will bring about a state of mental calm.
- Practising the forms involves balance, alignment, fine-scale motor control, rhythm of movement, and the genesis of movement from the body's vital centre.
- Proponents of tai chi believe that it improves walking and running. Many practitioners notice benefits in terms of correcting poor postural alignment or movement patterns that can contribute to tension or injury.
- The meditative nature of the exercises is calming and relaxing.
- Patient reports suggest that the practice of tai chi may improve balance and reduce falls.
- There is little scientific evidence supporting the practice of tai chi in improving symptoms of PD.

Dietary supplements

- The US National Institute of Health (NIH) Office of Dietary Supplements defines a dietary supplement as a product that:
  - ◇ Is intended to supplement the diet.
  - ◇ Contains one or more dietary ingredients (including vitamins, minerals, herbs or other botanicals, amino acids, and other substances) or their constituents.
  - ◇ Is intended to be taken by mouth as a pill, capsule, tablet, or liquid.
  - ◇ Is labelled on the front panel as being a dietary supplement.
- The Office of Dietary Supplements cautions that published analyses of herbal supplements have found differences between ingredients listed on the label and actual ingredients. The word 'standardized' on a product label is no guarantee of higher product quality, since in the USA there is no legal definition of 'standardized' (or 'certified' or 'verified') for supplements.
- There is little scientific evidence to support most of the following substances that are marked for the treatment of PD. Further testing is needed.

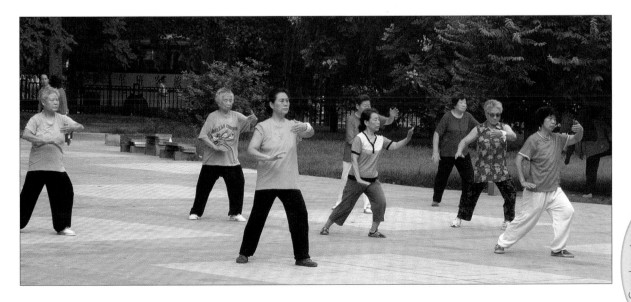

136 **Tai chi.** Elderly Chinese practise tai chi early in the morning in a Beijing park. *Photo courtesy of Mark J. Kingsley.*

Complementary medicine and Parkinson's disease

Coenzyme Q10

- CoQ10 is an antioxidant and a component of the energy-producing electron transport chain of mitochondria.
- It is currently being investigated as a neuro-protective agent.
- A double-blind, placebo-controlled pilot study in PD found that high doses of CoQ10 (1200 mg/day) were associated with a reduced rate of deterioration in motor function from baseline over 16 months. This result should be considered preliminary and further studies will be required.
- A futility study, sponsored by the NIH, is currently under way. Researchers are investigating doses of CoQ10 as high as 2400 mg/day.
- Tested formulations have usually included vitamin E (as did the placebo).
- Use of CoQ10 is usually not covered by insurance and high doses are relatively expensive.

Vitamin E

- Vitamin E is an antioxidant.
- Observational studies suggested that vitamin E may have a neuroprotective effect on decreasing the risk of Parkinson's disease.
- Zhang et al. (2002) evaluated the incidence of PD in two large cohorts of men and women who completed detailed and validated semiquantitative food frequency questionnaires. A total of 371 incident PD cases were ascertained in the Nurses' Health Study, which comprised 76,890 women who were followed for 14 years, and the Health Professionals Follow-Up Study, which comprised 47,331 men who were followed for 12 years. They found that neither intake of total vitamins E or C nor use of vitamin E or vitamin C supplements or multivitamins was significantly associated with decreased risk of PD. The risk of PD, however, was significantly reduced among men and women with high intake of dietary vitamin E from foods only.
- The DATATOP study (1993) found that vitamin E in doses of 2,000 IU did not delay the need for levodopa treatment in patients with early PD.
- A meta-analysis by Miller et al. (2005) of 19 clinical trials found that high-dosage vitamin E supplementation (400 IU/day for at least 1 year) may increase all-cause mortality. Benefits or risks of lower-dosage supplementation were unclear.

Glutathione

- Glutathione (GSH) is an antioxidant and an essential cofactor for antioxidant enzymes (**137**).
- It provides protection for mitochondria against endogenous oxygen radicals.
- Several studies have demonstrated a deficiency of reduced GSH in the substantia nigra of patients with PD.
- GSH is not well absorbed in an oral formulation.
- Sechi et al. (1996) studied the effects of GSH in nine patients with early, untreated PD in an open-label study. GSH was administered intravenously, 600 mg twice daily for 30 days. All patients were reported to improve significantly after GSH therapy, with a 42% decline in disability. Once GSH was stopped the therapeutic effect lasted for 2–4 months.
- There are no published double-blind, placebo-controlled clinical trials.
- A double-blind, placebo-controlled pilot study is currently under way at the Parkinson's Disease and Movement Disorders Center at the University of South Florida.
- Use of GSH is usually not covered by insurance and is relatively expensive.

Dehydroepiandrosterone

- Dehydroepiandrosterone (DHEA) is an endogenous hormone.
- DHEA levels in the body begin to decrease after the age of 30.
- DHEA can cause higher than normal levels of androgens and oestrogens in the body, and theoretically may increase the risk of prostate, breast, ovarian, and other hormone-sensitive cancers.
- Some research suggests that increasing oestrogen may be beneficial by modulating brain neurotransmitters or through possible neuroprotective activity. This has yet to be proven.

Curcumin (turmeric)

- Curcumin is an antioxidant derived from the curry spice turmeric.
- It may be an inducer of the heat shock response.
- It may provide an alternative, nutritional approach to reduce oxidative damage and amyloid pathology.
- There are no data available for treatment of PD.

137 Glutathione oxidation–reduction cycle.
Glutathione plays an important role in the scavenging of free radicals, such as hydrogen peroxide, which can damage cell metabolism. One molecule of hydrogen peroxide is reduced to two molecules of water, while two molecules of reduced glutathione (GSH) are oxidized to form GSSG. The enzymes which catalyse the redox reactions – glutathione peroxidase and glutathione reductase – are dependent on the presence of selenium and riboflavin (flavin adenine dinucleotide), respectively.

Chelation therapy

◆ Chelation therapy removes heavy metals from the body.
◆ Rare side-effects may include fever, headache, nausea, vomiting, a sudden drop in blood pressure, abnormally low calcium levels in the blood, permanent kidney damage, and bone marrow depression (meaning that blood cell counts fall).
◆ Reversible injury to the kidneys, although infrequent, has been reported with ethylenediamine tetra-acetic acid (EDTA) chelation therapy.
◆ There is no scientific evidence to support its use in PD.
◆ It is frequently recommended as a treatment following hair analysis, but this does not justify its use in PD (see below).

Hair analysis
◆ There are many web pages offering hair analysis as a way of diagnosing heavy metal exposure.
◆ Scientific studies demonstrate that this method is very unreliable.
◆ External contaminants, such as dust, shampoo, conditioners, or hair spray, influence the results.
◆ Frequently, the results are purported to indicate the need for additional treatment such as chelation therapy.
◆ Hair analysis should not be used to diagnose or treat heavy metal exposure in PD.

Enhanced external counterpulsation

◆ Enhanced external counterpulsation (EECP) is the sequential diastolic inflation of lower extremity pneumatic cuffs to augment aortic diastolic pressure, increase venous return to the heart, and decrease left ventricular afterload.
◆ It is an approved treatment for angina.
◆ Recently, web pages have begun offering EECP as a treatment for PD.
◆ Treatments are prescribed for 1 hr/day, 5 days a week, for 6 weeks.
◆ No scientific evidence supports its use.
◆ It is not covered by insurance and requires multiple treatments.

Resources

National support organizations

Australia
Parkinson's Australia Inc
Frewin Centre, Frewin Place
Scullin
ACT - 2614
t: (02) 6278 8916
e: norman.marshall@parkinsonsaustralia.
org.au
w: www.parkinsons.org.au

Brazil
Parkinson's Society—Rio de Janeiro
Rua Djalma Ulrich 163/906
22071-020
Rio de Janeiro
t: +359 2 989 0289
f: +359 2 971 3674
e: wbossnev_ams@yahoo.com

Associação Brasil Parkinson
Av. Bosque da Saude
1.155 – Sao Paulo
t/f: 011 578 8177
e: asparkin@netway.com.br
w: www.parkinson.org.br

Canada
Parkinson Society Canada
4211 Yonge Street
316 Toronto
ON M2P 2A9
t: + 416-227-9700
free: 1-800-565-3000 (National)
f: + 416-227-9600
e: general.info@parkinson.ca
w: www.parkinson.ca

Czech Republic
Young Czech Parkins
e: pavel.kner@email.cz
w: www.parkinson-cz.net

Denmark
Dansk Parkinsonforening
Kirke Værløsevej 26-1
Værløse 3500
t: +45 39 27 15 55
f: +45 39 18 20 75
e: dansk@parkinson.dk
w: www.parkinson.dk

Finland
Suomen Parkinson-liittory
The Finnish Parkinson Association
Erityisosaamiskeskus Suvituuli
(Rehabilitation Centre)
Suvilinnantie 2
PL 905
Turku 20101
t1: +358 2 2740 400 (Finnish)
t2: +358 2 2740 444 (English)
f: +358 2 2740 444
e: Parkinson-liitto@parkinson.fi
w: www.parkinson.fi

Germany
Deutsche Parkinson Vereinigung
Bundesverband e.V.
Mehrhoff
Moselstraße 31
41464 Neuss
t: 02131/740 270
f: 02131/4 54 45
e: info@parkinson-vereinigung.de
w: www.parkinson-vereinigung.de

India
Parkinson's Disease Foundation of India
Jaslok Hospital and Research Center
Pedder Road, Mumbai-400 026.
t: 5664 0302, 5657 3230
f: 2352 1458
e: drbhatt@hotmail.com
w: parkinsonsdiseaseindia.com

Japan
Japanese Parkinson's Disease Association
1-9-13-812
Akasaka
Minato-ku
Tokyo
t: 03 3560 3355
f: 03 3560 3356
e: jpda@mud.biglobe.ne.jp

Malaysia
Persatuan Parkinson Malaysia
Malaysian Parkinson's Disease Association
35 Jalan Nyaman 10
Happy Garden
58200 Kuala Lumpur
t: 03 7980 6685
f: 03 7982 6685
e: mpda1@streamyx.com
w: www.mpda.org.my

Netherlands
ParkinsonPlaza
P.O. Box 67
AB 6680, Bemmel
t: +31 481 465294
f: +31 481 461243
e: info@parkinsonplaza.nl
w: www.parkinsonplaza.nl

New Zealand
Parkinsons Auckland
P.O. Box 16-238
7a Taylors Road
Sandringham
Auckland
t: 09 278 6918
free: 0800 000 408 (National)
e: aklparkinsons@xtra.co.nz
w: www.parkinsonsauckland.org.nz

Pakistan
Pakistan Parkinson's Society (PPS)
67-1, 3rd Street,
Kh Badban, Phase V
DHA
Karachi 75500
t: +92300 8220196
e: pakistanparkinsonssociety
@yahoo.com
w: www.parkinsons.org.pk

Portugal
Associação Portuguesa de Doentes de
Parkinson (APDPk)
José Luís Mota Vieira
Rua Frei Manuel do Sepilcro, 26,
R/C 8500-680 Portimão
Algarve
Delegação do Algarve
[Algarve Parkinson Branch – Portugal]
t: 36 1 455 5819
f: 36 1 455 5819
e: parkinsonalgarve@clix.pt
w: www.parkinson.pt

Singapore
Parkinson's Disease Society (Singapore)
c/o NNI Administration, Level 2
National Neuroscience Institute 11
Jalan Tan Tock Seng
Singapore 308433
t: (65) 6357 7060
f: (65) 6256 4755
e: pds@nni.com.sg
w: www.parkinsonsingapore.com

Spain
Asociación Parkinson Internet
Apanet
Calle Collado de Marichiva 3
3A 28035 Madrid
Spain
t: 902 502 603
e: parkinson@apanet.org.es
w: www.apanet.org.es

Sweden
ParkinsonFörbundet
The Swedish Parkinson's Disease
Association
Box 1386
Sundbyberg 17227
t: +46 8 546 405 27
e: parkinsonforbundet.kansli@telia.com
w: www.parkinsonforbundet.se

Taiwan
Taiwan Parkinson Association
c/o Department of Neurology
National Taiwan University Hospital
No 7 Chung-shan South Road
Taipei 100
t: 886 2 23123456 ext 5343
f: 886 2 23418395

UK
Parkinson's Disease Society
National Office
215 Vauxhall Bridge Road,
London, SW1V 1EJ
t: 020 7931 8080
f: 020 7233 9908 / 020 7963 9360
e: enquiries@parkinsons.org.uk
w: www.parkinsons.org.uk

European Parkinson's Disease Association
(EPDA)
4 Golding Road,
Sevenoaks, Kent, TN13 3NJ
t/f: 01732 457 683
e: lizzie@epda.eu.com

The National Tremor Foundation
Disablement Services Centre
Harold Wood Hospital,
Gubbins Lane,
Harold Wood,
Romford, Essex, RM3 OAR
t: 0800 3288046
f: 01708 378032
e: tremorfoundation@aol.com

The Sarah Matheson Trust
for Multiple System Atrophy
Pickering Unit, St Mary's Hospital,
London W2 1NY
t: 020 7886 1520
e: office@msaweb.co.uk
w: www.tremor.org.uk
w: www.msaweb.co.uk

The PSP Association
The Old Rectory
Wappenham
Towcester
Northants, NN12 8SQ
t: 01327 860299
e: psp@pspeur.org
w: www.pspeur.org

USA
National Parkinson Foundation, Inc.
1501 N.W. 9th Avenue/Bob Hope Road
Miami, Florida 33136-1494
t: 305 2436666
free: 1 800 327 4545
f: 305 243 5595
w: www.parkinson.org

International Essential Tremor Foundation
P.O. Box 14005
Lenexa, Kansas 66285-4005
t: 913 341 3880
f: 913 341 1296
free: 888 387 3667
e: staff@essentialtremor.org

Society for Progressive Supranuclear Palsy
Executive Plaza III
11350 McCormick Road, Suite 906
Hunt Valley, MD 21031
t: 800 457 4777
f: 410 785 7009
w: www.psp.org

APDA National Office,
1250 Hylan Blvd., Suite 4B
Staten Island, NY 10305
t: 1-800-223-2732
f: 1-718-981-4399
e: apda@apdaparkinson.org
w: www.apdaparkinson.org

Shy-Drager/Multiple System Atrophy
Support Group, Inc.
P.O. Box 279
Coupland, TX 78615
t: 866 SDS 4999 (737 4999)
f: 512 251 3315
e: Don.Summers@shy-drager.com
w: www.shy-drager.com

Physical/occupational therapy resources

The National Center on Physical Activity
and Disability www.ncpad.com

American Physical Therapy Association
www.apta.org

The Chartered Society of Physiotherapy
www.csp.org.uk

The College of Occupational Therapists
www.cot.org.uk/

Patient support programmes

Bristol-Myers Squibb Patient Assistance
Foundation, Inc.,
P.O. Box 1058, Somerville, NJ 08876
t: 1 800 736 0003
f: 1 800 736 1611.

GlaxoSmithKline Bridges to Access
PO Box 29038, Phoenix, AZ 85038-9038,

Together Rx Access Card is sponsored by
several of the world's pharmaceutical
companies: Abbott Laboratories;
AstraZeneca; Bristol-Myers Squibb
Company; GlaxoSmithKline; Janssen
Pharmaceutica Products, L.P.; LifeScan,
a Johnson & Johnson company; Novartis
Pharmaceuticals Corporation; Ortho-
McNeil Pharmaceutical, Inc.; Pfizer Inc.;
Sanofi-Aventis; Takeda Pharmaceuticals
North America, Inc.; and TAP
Pharmaceutical Products Inc.
Together Rx Access LLC, PO Box 9426,
Wilmington, DE 19809-994

Wyeth Pharmaceutical Assistance
Foundation
P.O. Box 1759, Paoli, PA 19301-0859
t: 1 800 568 9938

Dietician resources

Hip Savers
1-800-358-4477 or 781-828-3880
http://www.hipsavers.com/index.html
hipsavers@msn.com

Dietary Approaches to Stop Hypertension
(DASH)
http://www.nhlbi.nih.gov/health/public
/heart/hbp/dash/new_dash.pdf
http://www.nih.gov/news/pr/apr97/
Dash.htm
http://www.nhlbi.nih.gov/hbp/prevent/
h_eating/h_e_dash.htm
http://www.cspinet.org/nah/dashdiet.
htm
http://www.mckinley.uiuc.edu/health-
info/dis-cond/bloodpr/dash-1500.html

Literature
*Parkinson's Disease: Guidelines for
Medical Nutrition Therapy.* Professional
manual in binder form.

*Eat Well, Stay Well With Parkinson's
Disease.* For patients and families.

Parkinson's Disease and Constipation.
Audiotape and guidebook for patients,
families, and group use.

All from: Five Star Living, 1409 Olive Ct.,
Unit E, Ft. Collins, CO 80524.

Further reading

Chapter 1

Ben Shlomo Y (1997) The epidemiology of Parkinson's disease. *Baillieres Clinical Neurology and Neurosurgery* 6:55–68.

Braak H, Del Tredici K, Rub U *et al.* (2003) Staging of brain pathology related to sporadic Parkinson's disease. *Neurobiology of Ageing* 24:197–211.

Di Monte DA, Lavasani M, Manning-Bog AB (2002) Environmental factors in Parkinson's disease. *Neurotoxicology* 23:487–502.

Morris HR (2005) Genetics of Parkinson's disease. *Annals of Medicine* 37:86–96.

Chapter 2

Calne DB, Snow BJ, Lee C (1992) Criteria for diagnosing Parkinson's disease. *Annals of Neurology* 32(suppl):S125–S127.

Gelb DJ, Oliver E, Gilman S (1999) Diagnostic criteria for Parkinson's disease. *Archives of Neurology* 56:33–39.

Hughes AJ, Daniel SE, Blankson S, Lees AJ (1993) A clinicopathologic study of 100 cases of Parkinson's disease. *Archives of Neurology* 50:140–148.

Hughes AJ, Daniel SE, Lees AJ (2001) Improved accuracy of clinical diagnosis of Lewy body Parkinson's disease. *Neurology* 57:1497–1499.

Nutt JG, Wooten GF (2005) Clinical Practice. Diagnosis and initial management of Parkinson's disease. *The New England Journal of Medicine* 353:1021–1027.

Chapter 3

Clarke CE, Davies P (2000) Systematic review of acute levodopa and apomorphine challenge tests in the diagnosis of idiopathic Parkinson's disease. *Journal of Neurology, Neurosurgery and Psychiatry* 69:590–594.

Fischman AJ (2005) Role of [18F]-dopa PET imaging in assessing movement disorders. *Radiology Clinics of North America* 43:93–106.

Marshall V, Grosset D (2003) Role of dopamine transporter imaging in routine clinical practice. *Movement Disorders* 18:1415–1423.

Chapter 4

Parkinson's Study Group (2002) A controlled trial of rasagiline in early Parkinson's disease: The TEMPO study. *Archives of Neurology* 59(12):1937–1943.

Parkinson's Study Group (2005) A randomised placebo-controlled trial of rasagiline in levodopa-treated patients with Parkinson's disease and motor fluctuations: the PRESTO study. *Archives of Neurology* 62(2):241–248.

Rascol O, Brooks DJ, Melamed E *et al.* (2005) Rasagiline as an adjunct to levodopa in patients with Parkinson's disease and motor fluctuations (LARGO, Lasting effect in Adjuct therapy with Rasagiline Given Once Daily study): a randomised, double-blind, parallel-group trial. *Lancet* 365(9643):947–954.

Chapter 5

Appenzeller O, Gross JE (1971) Autonomic deficits in Parkinson's syndrome. *Archives of Neurology* 24:50–57.

Comella C, Tanner C, Ristanovic R (1993) Polysomnographic sleep measures in Parkinson's disease patients with treatment-induced hallucinations. *Annals of Neurology* 34:710–714.

Comella CL (2003) Sleep disturbances in Parkinson's disease. *Current Neurology and Neuroscience Reports* 3:173–180.

Cummings JL (1991) Behavioral complications of drug treatment of Parkinson's disease. *Journal of the American Geriatrics Society* 39:708–716.

Cummings JL (1992) Depression and Parkinson's disease: a review. *American Journal of Psychiatry* 149:443–454.

Daniele A, Albanese A, Contarino MF *et al.* (2003) Cognitive and behavioural effects of chronic stimulation of the subthalamic nucleus in patients with Parkinson's disease. *Journal of Neurology, Neurosurgery and Psychiatry* 74(2):175–182.

Fernandez HH, Trieschmann ME, Okun MS (2005) Rebound psychosis: effect of discontinuation of antipsychotics in Parkinson's disease. *Movement Disorders* 20(1):104–105.

Fernandez HH, Trieschmann ME, Friedman JH (2004) Aripiprazole for drug induced psychosis in Parkinson's disease; preliminary experience. *Clinical Neuropharmacology* 27:4–5.

Fernandez HH, Trieschmann ME, Burke MA *et al.* (2003) Long-term quetiapine use for drug-induced psychosis among parkinsonian patients. *Movement Disorders* 18(5):510–514.

Fernandez HH, Trieschmann ME, Friedman JH (2003) The treatment of psychosis in Parkinson's disease: safety considerations. *Drug Safety* 26(9):643–659.

Fernandez HH, Friedman JH, Jacques C, Rosenfield M (1999) Quetiapine for the treatment of drug-induced psychosis in Parkinson's disease. *Movement Disorders* 14(3):484–487.

Fernandez HH, Friedman JH. (1999) Punding on L-dopa. *Movement Disorders* 14(5):836–838.

Fernandex HH, Simuni T (2005) Anxiety in Parkinson's disease. In: *Parkinson's Disease and Nonmotor Dysfunction.* RF Pfeiffer, I Bodis-Wolllner (eds.) The Humana Press, Totowa, New Jersey, pp. 13–23.

Fernandez HH and Shinobu L (2004) Dementia and psychosis. In: *Therapy of Parkinson's Disease: Third Edition.* R Pahwa, K Lyons, W Holler (eds.) Marcel Dekker, New York, pp. 391–423.

Ford B, Lynch T, Greene P (1994) Risperidone in Parkinson's Disease. *Lancet* 344:681.

Friedman JH, Fernandez HH (2000) Non-motor problems in Parkinson's disease. *Neurology* 6(1):18–27.

Frucht S, Rogers JD, Greene PE *et al.* (1999) Falling asleep at the wheel: motor vehicle mishaps in persons taking pramipexole and ropinirole. *Neurology* **52**:1908–1910.

Goetz CG, Poewe W, Rascol O, Sampaio C (2005) Evidence-based medical review update: pharmacological and surgical treatments of Parkinson's disease: 2001–2004. *Movement Disorders* **20**(5):523–539.

Gotham AM, Brown RG, Marsden CD (1986) Depression in Parkinson's disease: a quantitative and qualitative analysis. *Journal of Neurology, Neurosurgery and Psychiatry* **49**:381–389.

Gschwandtner U, Aston J, Renaud S, Fuhr P (2001) Pathologic gamblilng in patients with Parkinson's disease. *Clinical Neuropharmacology* **24**:170–172.

Hiner BC (2000) Autonomic complications of Parkinson's disease. In: *Parkinson's Disease and Movement Disorders.* CH Adler, JE Ahlskog (eds.) Human Press, Totowa, New Jersey, pp. 161–174.

Molina JA, Sainz-Artiga MJ, Fraile A *et al.* (2000) Pathologic gambling in Parkinson's disease: a behavioral manifestation of pharmacologic treatment? *Movement Disorders* **15**:869–872.

Nausieda P, Weiner W, Kaplan L *et al.* (1982) Sleep disruption in the course of chronic levodopa therapy: an early feature of levodopa psychosis. *Clinical Neuropharmacology* **5**:183–194.

Ravina B, Putt M, Siderowf A *et al.* (2005) Donepezil in Parkinson's disease: a randomized, double-blind, placebo-controlled, crossover study. *Journal of Neurology, Neurosurgery and Psychiatry* **76**(7):934–939.

Rich SS, Freidman JH, Ott BR (1995) Risperidone versus clozapine in the treatment of psychosis in six patients with Parkinson's disease and other akinetic-rigid syndromes. *Journal of Clinical Psychiatry* **56**(12):556–559.

Saint-Cyr JA, Trepanier LL, Kumar R *et al.* (2000) Neuropsychological consequences of chronic bilateral stimulation of the subthalamic nucleus in Parkinson's disease. *Brain* **123**(10):2091–2108.

Starkstein SE, Robinson RG, Leiguarda R (1993) Anxiety and depression in Parkinson's disease. *Behavioural Neurology* **6**:151–154.

Stein M, Heuser IJ, Juncos JL, Uhde TW (1990) Anxiety disorders in patients with Parkinson's disease. *American Journal of Psychiatry* **147**:217–220.

Wint DP, Okun MS, Fernandex HH (2004) Psychosis in Parkinson's disease. *Journal of Geriatric Psychiatry and Neurology* **17**(3):127–136.

Zesiewicz TA, Baker MJ, Wahba M, Hauser RA (2003) Autonomic nervous system dysfunction in Parkinson's disease. *Current Treatment Options in Neurology* **5**:149–160.

Zoldan J, Friedberg G, Goldberg-Stern H, Melamed E (1993) Odansetron for hallucinosis in advanced Parkinson's disease. *Lancet* **341**:562–563.

Chapter 6

Chaudhuri KR, Pal S, DiMarco A *et al.* (2002) The Parkinson's disease sleep scale: a new instrument for assessing sleep and nocturnal disability in Parkinson's disease. *Journal of Neurology, Neurosurgery and Psychiatry* **73**:629–635.

Chaudhuri KR, Martinez-Martin P, Schapira AH *et al.* (2006) International multicenter pilot study of the first comprehensive self-completed non-motor symptoms questionnaire for Parkinson's disease: the NMSQuest study. *Movement Disorders* **21**(7):916–923.

Cummings JL, Mega M, Gray K *et al.* (1994) The Neuropsychiatric Inventory: comprehensive assessment of psychopathology in dementia. *Neurology* **44**:2308–2314.

Folstein MF, Folstein SE, McHugh PR (1975) Mini-Mental State: a practical method for grading the cognitive state of patients for the clinician. *Journal of Psychiatric Research* **12**:189–198.

Friedberg G, Zoldan J, Weizman A, Melamed E (1998) Parkinson Psychosis Rating Scale: a practical instrument for grading psychosis in Parkinson's disease. *Clinical Neuropharmcology* **21**:280–284.

Goetz CG, Stebbins GT, Chmura TA *et al.* (1995) Teaching tape for the motor section of the unified Parkinson's disease rating scale. *Movement Disorders* **10**(3):263–266.

Goetz CG, Poewe R, Rascol O *et al.* (2004) Movement Disorder Society Task Force on Rating Scales for Parkinson's Disease. Movement Disorder Society Task Force report on the Hoehn and Yahr staging scale: status and recommendations. *Movement Disorders* **19**:1020–1028.

Hamilton M (1967) Development of a rating scale for primary depressive illness. *British Journal of Social and Clinical Psychology* **6**:278–296.

Hauser RA, Friedlander J, Zesiewicz TA *et al.* (2000) A home diary to assess functional status in patients with Parkinson's disease with motor fluctuations and dyskinesia. *Clinical Neuropharmacology* **23**:75–81.

Hoehn MM, Yahr MD (1967) Parkinsonism: onset, progression and mortality. *Neurology* **17**:427–442.

Johns MW (1991) A new method for measuring daytime sleepiness: the Epworth Sleepiness Scale. *Sleep* **14**:540–545.

Levin BE, Llabre MM, Weiner WJ (1988) Parkinson's disease and depression: psychometric properties of the Beck Depression Inventory. *Journal of Neurology, Neurosurgery and Psychiatry* **51**:1401–1404.

Mattis S (1988) *Dementia Rating Scale Professional Manual.* Psychological Assessment Resources, Odessa.

Movement Disorder Society Task Force on Rating Scales for Parkinson's Disease (2003) The Unified Parkinson's Disease Rating Scale (UPDRS); status and recommendations. *Movement Disorders* **18**:738–750.

Okun MS, Fernandez HH, Pedraza O (2004) Development and initial validation of a screening tool for Parkinson's Disease surgical candidates. *Neurology* **63**:161–163.

Overall JE, Gorham DR (1962) The Brief Psychiatric Rating Scale. *Psychological Reports* **10**:799–812.

Peto V, Jenkinson C, Fitzpatrick R, Greenhall R (1995) The development and validation of a short measure of functioning and well-being for individuals with Parkinson's disease. *Quality of Life Research* **4**:241–248.

Psychopharmacology Research Branch, NIMH 1976 Abnormal Involuntary Movement Scale (AIMS). In: *EDCEU Assessment Manual for Psychopharmacology*, revised DHEW Pub No (ADM) 76-338. Guy W (ed.) National Institute of Mental Health, Rockville, Maryland, pp. 534–537.

Ramaker C, Marinus J, Stiggelbout AM, Van Hilten BJ (2002) Systematic evaluation of rating scales for impairment and disability in Parkinson's disease. *Movement Disorders* **17**:867–876.

Yesavage J, Brink T, Rose T *et al.* (1983) Development and validation of a geriatric depression screening scale: a preliminary report. *Journal of Psychiatric Research* 17:37–49.

Chapter 7

Krack P, Fraix V, Mendes A *et al.* (2002) Postoperative management of subthalamic nucleus stimulation for Parkinson's disease. *Movement Disorders* 17(suppl 3):S188–S197.

Vitek JL, Bakay RA, Hashimoto T *et al.* (1998) Microelectrode-guided pallidotomy: technical approach and its application in medically intractable Parkinson's disease. *Journal of Neurosurgery* 88(6):1027–1043.

Okun MS, Green J, Saben R *et al.* (2003) Mood changes with deep brain stimulation of STN and GPi: results of a pilot study. *Journal of Neurology, Neurosurgery and Psychiatry* 74(11):1584–1586.

Okun MS, Fernandez HH, Pedraza O *et al.* (2004) Development and initial validation of a screening tool for Parkinson's disease surgical candidates. *Neurology* 63(1):161–163.

Okun MS, Vitek JL (2004) Lesion therapy for Parkinson's disease and other movement disorders: update and controversies. *Movement Disorders* 19(4):375–389.

Romrell J, Fernandez HH, Okun MS (2003) Rationale for current therapies in Parkinson's disease. *Expert Opinion on Pharmacotherapy* 4(10):1747–1761.

Saint-Cyr JA, Trepanier LL, Kumar R *et al.* (2000) Neuropsychological consequences of chronic bilateral stimulation of the subthalamic nucleus in Parkinson's disease. *Brain* 123(10):2091–2108.

Chapter 8

Jarman B, Hurwitz B, Cook A *et al.* (2002) Effects of community based nurses specialising in Parkinson's disease on health outcome and costs: randomised controlled trial. *British Medical Journal* 324(7345):1072–1075.

MacMahon D (1999) Parkinson's disease nurse specialist: an important role in disease management. *Neurology* 527(suppl 3):S21–S25.

Raynolds H, Wilson Barnett J, Richardson G (2000) Evaluation of the role of the Parkinson's disease nurse specialist. *International Journal of Nursing Studies* 37(4):337–349.

Taft JM, Hooker RS (1999) Physician assistants in neurology practice. *Neurology* 52(7):1513.

Taft JM, Hooker RS (2000) Physician assistants and the practice of neurology. *Journal of the American Academy of Physician Assistants* 17(2):55–56.

Young C, Abercrombie M, Beattie A (2003) How a specialist nurse helps patients undergoing deep brain stimulation. *Professional Nurse* 18(6):318–321.

Chapter 9

American Physical Therapy Association (2003) *Guide to Physical Therapist Practice*, 2nd edn. American Physical Therapy Association, Alexandria.

Argue J (2000) *Parkinson's Disease and the Art of Moving*. New Harbinger Publications, Oakland, California.

Byl NN, Melnick ME (1997) The neural consequences of repetition: Clinical implications of a learning hypothesis. *Journal of Hand Therapy* 10:160–172.

Clapcich J, Goldberg N, Walsh E (1999) *Be independent!: A self-help guide for people with Parkinson's disease.* American Parkinson's Disease Association, Staten Island, New York.

Cornhill M (1996) In-hand manipulation: The association to writing skills. *American Journal of Occupational Therapy* 50:732–739.

Gaudet P (2002) Measuring the impact of Parkinson's disease: An occupational therapy perspective. *Canadian Journal of Occupational Therapy* 69:104–113.

Gauthier L, Dalziel S, Gauthie S (1987) The benefits of group occupational therapy for patients with Parkinson's disease. *American Journal of Occupational Therapy* 41(6):360–365.

Karlson K, Larson J, Tandberg E, Maeland J (1999) Influences of clinical and demographic variables in quality of life in patients with Parkinson's disease. *Journal of Neurology, Neuropsychiatry and Psychiatry* 66:431–435.

Laufer L (2004) *Handwriting Exercises to Music: Callirobics.* Box 6634, Charlottesville, Virginia.

Morris ME (2000) Movement disorders in people with Parkinson's disease: a model for physical therapy. *Physical Therapy* 80:578–597.

Murphy S, Tickle-Degnen L (2001) The effectiveness of occupational therapy-related treatments for persons with Parkinson's disease: A meta-analytic review. *American Journal of Occupational Therapy* 55(4):385–392.

Pedretti LW (1996) *Occupational Therapy Practice Skills for Physical Dysfunction*, 4th edn. Mosby, St. Louis, Missouri.

Petro V, Jenkinson C, Fitzpatrick R (1995) The development and validation of a short measure of functioning and well being for individuals with Parkinson's disease. *Quality of Life Research* 4:241–248.

Schneider JS, Diamond SG, Markham CH (1987) Parkinson's disease: sensory and motor problems in arms and hands. *Neurology* 37:954–960.

Trombly C, Radomski M (2002) *Occupational Therapy for Physical Dysfunction*, 5th edn. Lipincott Williams and Wilkins, Philaldelphia.

Umphred DA (2001) *Neurological Rehabilitation*, 4th edn. Mosby, St. Louis, Missouri.

Chapter 10

Beukelman DR, Yorkston KM, Reichle J (2000) *Augmentative and Alternative Communication for Adults with Acquired Neurologic Disorders.* Paul H Brookes Publishing, Baltimore, Maryland.

Castell JA, Johnston BT, Colcher A *et al.* (2001) Manometric abnormalities of the oesophagus in patients with Parkinson's disease. *Neurogastroenterology and Motility* 13:361–364.

Crossan B (1992) *Subcortical Functions in Language and Memory.* The Guilford Press, New York.

Darley FL, Aronson AE, Brown JR (1975) *Motor Speech Disorders.* WB Saunders, Philadelphia.

Duffy JR (2005) *Motor Speech Disorders*, 2nd edn. Yearbook, St. Louis, Missouri.

Ho AK, Bradshaw JL, Iansek R, Alfredson R (1999) Speech volume regulation in Parkinson's disease: effects of implicit cues and explicit instructions. *Neuropsychologia* 37:1453–1460.

Krack P, Poepping M, Weinert D *et al.* (2000) Thalamic, pallidal, or subthalamic surgery for Parkinson's disease? *Journal of Neurology* 247:122–134.

Miller AJ (1999) *The Neuroscientific Principles of Swallowing and Dysphagia.* Singular Publishing Group, San Diego.

Miller RM, Groher ME (1997) General treatment of neurologic swallowing disorders. In: *Dysphagia: Diagnosis and Management*, 3rd edn. ME Groher (ed.) Butterworth-Heinemann, Boston, pp. 223–243.

Murray J, Musson N (2005) *Understanding dysphagia* (Version 1.0) [CDROM]. (Available from the North Florida Foundation for Research and Education, Inc., Gainesville, FL).

Nilsson H, Ekberg O, Olsson R, Hindfelt B (1996) Quantitative assessment of oral and pharyngeal function in Parkinson's disease. *Dysphagia* 11:144–150.

Ramig LO, Brin MF, Velickovic M, Fox C (2004) Hypokinetic laryngeal movement disrders. In: *The MIT Encyclopedia of Communication Disorders*. RD Kent (ed.). The Massachusetts Institute of Technology Press, Cambridge, Massachusetts, pp. 30–32.

Rosenbek JC, Jones H N (2007). Dysphagia in patients with motor speech disorders. In: *Motor speech disorders*, G. Weismer (ed.) Plural Publishing, San Diego, pp. 221–259.

Rosenbek JC, LaPointe LL (1985) In: *Clinical Management of Neurogenic Communicative Disorders*, 2nd edn. DF Johns (ed.) Little, Brown, pp. 97–152.

Santens P, De Letter M, Van Borsel J *et al.* (2003) Lateralized effects of subthalamic nucleus stimulation on different aspects of speech in Parkinson's disease. *Brain and Language* 87:253–258.

Schulz GM, Grant MK (2000) Effects of speech therapy and pharmacologic and surgical treatments on voice and speech in Parkinson's disease: A review of the literature. *Journal of Communication Disorders* 33:59–88.

Yorkston KM, Beukelman DR, Strand EA, Bell KR (1999) *Management of Motor Speech Disorders in Children and Adults*. Pro-Ed, Austin, Texas.

Yorkston KM, Miller RM, Strand EA (1995) *Management of Speech and Swallowing in Degenerative Diseases*. Communication Skill Builders, San Antonio, Texas.

Chapter 11

See Resources section.

Chapter 12

Adams JD Jr, Klaidman LK, Odunze IN *et al.* (1991) Alzheimer's and Parkinson's disease. Brain levels of glutathione, glutathione disulfide, and vitamin E. *Molecular Clinical Neuropathology* 14:213–226.

Barrett S (2005) *Commercial Hair Analysis: A Cardinal Sign of Quackery*. Available: http://www.quackwatch.com/01QuackeryRelatedTopics/hair.html [cited 2 January 2005]

Barrett S (1985) Commercial hair analysis: science or scam? *Journal of the American Medical Association* 254:1041–1045.

Etminan M, Gill SS, Samii A (2005) Intake of vitamin E, vitamin C, and carotenoids and the risk of Parkinson's disease: a meta-analysis. *Lancet Neurology* 4(6):362–365.

Cyr M, Calon F, Morissette M *et al.* (2000) Drugs with estrogen-like potency and brain activity: potential therapeutic applications for the CNS. *Current Pharmaceutical Design* 6(12):1287–1312.

Forrelli T (2003) Understanding herb–drug interactions. *Techniques in Orthopaedics* 18(1):37–45.

Frumkin H, Manning CC, Williams PL *et al.* (2001) Diagnostic chelation challenge with DMSA: a biomarker of long-term mercury exposure? *Environmental Health Perspectives* 109:167–171.

Hu Z, Yang X, Ho P *et al.* (2005) Herb–drug interactions: a literature review. *Drugs* 65(9):1239–1282.

Jenner P (1994) Oxidative damage in neurodegenerative disease. *Lancet* 17:796–798.

Manyam BV, Sanchez-Ramos JR (1999) Traditional and complementary therapies in Parkinson's disease. *Advances in Neurology* 80:565–574.

Miller ER, Pastor-Barriuso R, Dalal D *et al.* (2005) Meta-analysis: high-dosage vitamin E supplementation may increase all-cause mortality. *Annals of Internal Medicine* 142(1):37–46.

Parkinson Study Group (1993) Effects of tocopherol and deprenyl on the progression of disability in early Parkinson's disease. *The New England Journal of Medicine* 328:176–183.

Rabinstein A, Shulman L (2003) Acupuncture in clinical neurology. *Neurologist* 9(3):137–148.

Rajendran PR, Thompson RE, Reich SG (2001) The use of alternative therapies by patients with Parkinson's disease. *Neurology* 57:790–794.

Sechi G, Deledda MG, Bua G *et al.* (1996) Reduced intravenous glutathione in the treatment of early Parkinson's disease. *Progress in Neuropsychopharmacology and Biological Psychiatry* 20(7):1159–1170.

Seidel S, Kreutzer R, Smith D *et al.* (2001) Assessment of commercial laboratories performing hair mineral analysis. *The Journal of the American Medical Association* 285:67–72.

Shulman LM, Wen X, Weiner WJ (2002) Acupuncture therapy for the symptoms of Parkinson's disease. *Movement Disorders* 17:799–802.

Shultz CW, Oakes D, Kieburtz K *et al.* (2002) Effects of coenzyme Q10 in early Parkinson's disease: evidence of slowing of the functional decline. *Archives of Neurology* 59:1541–1550.

Zhang SM, Hernan MA, Chen H *et al.* (2002) Intakes of vitamins E and C, carotenoids, vitamin supplements, and Parkinson's disease risk. Comments. *Neurology* 59(8):E8–9.

Glossary

[18F] fluorodopa A labelled marker of dopamine activity which localizes to the presynaptic neurones. Activity is reduced in PD.

Adenyl cyclase An enzyme which is widespread in human and animal cells and works with AMP and other chemicals to produce energy.

Agnosia Lack of knowledge for specific, usually higher neurological, functions. This usually occurs due to an inability to process information rather than damage to the primary structure.

Akinetic rigid A subtype of PD where the patient has little or no tremor and hence the bradykinesia or akinesia and rigidity are the dominant features.

Alpha-synuclein A protein found in the substantia nigra, thalamus, and other brain areas that is normally unstructured and soluble. In PD and other conditions in which there are Lewy bodies, alpha-synuclein forms insoluble fibrils which can be seen through a microscope.

Alzheimer's disease One of the commonest forms of dementia, in which there is premature mental deterioration typically involving memory and language.

AMP (adenosine monophosphate). A chemical found in human and animal cells which has a central role in energy production.

Aphasia/dysphasia Difficulty in speaking and/or understanding speech.

Apoptosis The process of cell death which is considered pre-programmed but has an intial trigger. (The exact triggers are not known but may include toxins.)

Arteriovenous malformation A collection of abnormal arteries and veins formed during early body development.

Atropine An anticholinergic drug derived from Solanaceae plants, which increases the heart rate, dilates the pupils, and reduces secretions such as saliva.

Axial symptoms Involvement of the trunk and neck, typically in a Parkinson condition. Predominant axial involvement is typical of progressive supranuclear palsy.

Basal ganglia A collection of nerve cell groupings situated at the base of the brain, which control body movement and other functions such as cognition and emotion. The individual nuclei that make up the basal ganglia are the striatum (which consists of the caudate and putamen), the globus pallidus, the subthalamic nucleus, and the substantia nigra.

Basal proencephalon The area of the brain at the front/lower end, also known as the forebrain, being the part of the cerebral cortex that contains the limbic system, which controls emotion and longer-term memory.

Blepharospasm An involuntary, fast blinking of the eyelids that can be part of Parkinson conditions such as progressive supranuclear palsy and corticobasal degeneration.

Braak hypothesis A description of the staging of PD, rising from the brainstem to the basal ganglia and progresssing upwards to the cerebral cortex.

Bradykinesia Slowness of movement typical of PD, specifically with progressive reduction in both speed and amplitude of movement. Other disorders, e.g. hypothyroidism or depression, may feature general slowness of movement, but this is not true bradykinesia.

Brainstem The lower part of the brain, sited below the balance centre and above the spinal cord. Crucial nerves controlling breathing and swallowing are situated here.

Caeruloplasmin A protein in the blood which carries copper. Caeruloplasmin levels are low in patients with Wilson's disease, resulting in damage to nerve cells and the liver and causing a rare form of parkinsonism.

Cardiac tamponade A serious heart condition in which fluid collects in the pericardium and may prevent blood flow around the body by pressing in on the heart.

Caudate One of the basal ganglia components which degenerates in PD. The caudate and putamen (together called the striatum) both suffer cell death in PD.

Central tegmental area/ventral tegmentum Part of the midbrain lying close to the red nucleus and substantia nigra. It is considered to be part of the 'reward circuit' involved in behavioural motivation.

Cerebral cortex The outer layer of the brain, also referred to as 'grey matter'. Specific areas or 'lobes' are responsible for thinking, initiating motor movement, feeling sensation, producing speech, and for special senses such as vision.

Cholinergic system A system of nerve cells which involve the chemical acetycholine. Overactivity of the cholinergic system results in tremor and underactivity results in memory impairment.

Cholinesterase inhibitors (or acetylcholinesterase inhibitors). These drugs increase the amount of choline and are used as a treatment for dementia, such as occurs with Alzheimer's disease and PD.

Chorea Involuntary movements featuring jumping or jerking, often with some rotation, in the limbs, head, or body. It is sometimes used to describe dyskinesia, as in levodopa-induced chorea.

Choreoathetosis An involuntary movement which involves rotation and jerky or jumpy movements.

Compartment syndrome Inflammation of the tissues, typically in the lower leg, resulting in high pressure which needs surgical release.

Compliance (or adherence). The extent to which the patient takes a dose of medication in relation to the dose which has been recommended by their physician.

Concordance A process of consultation between the patient and the healthcare professional over assesment and treatment options resulting in an agreed management programme.

Depersonalization /derealization An alteration in an individual's self-perception or experience of the environment characterized by feelings of detachment and unreality.

Dopa decarboxylase An enzyme which aids the conversion of levodopa to dopamine. It also has some function in the production of serotonin.

Dopamine A brain neurotransmitter which, among other functions, is responsible for helping promote movement. It is produced in several areas of the brain, including the substantia nigra and the ventral tegmental area. Dopamine deficiency is associated with PD; drug therapy to increase dopamine levels involves levodopa, which can cross the blood–brain barrier and is then converted into dopamine, rather than dopamine itself, which cannot.

Dopamine agonist A chemical which is similar in structure to dopamine and can function as a dopamine substitute.

Dopamine receptor A specialized site on the outer surface of a neurone which receives signals from (i.e. gets stimulated by) dopamine.

Dopamine receptor subtype There are five distinguishable types of dopamine receptor (D1, D2, D3, D4, and D5) within the nervous system.

Dopamine transporter A carrier system for recycling dopamine within the synaptic cleft from the post-synaptic to the pre-synaptic neurone.

Dopaminergic Relating to, or activated by dopamine. The term can also be applied to drug treatments which replace deficient dopamine.

Dorsal motor nuclei A collection of nuclei in the posterior (dorsal) part of the brainstem that are the control centres for movements of the face and swallowing.

Dysautonomia Abnormality of function of the autonomic nervous system typically resulting in postural hypotension, bladder, bowel and sweating disturbance.

Dyskinesia Abnormal involuntary movement typical of more advanced PD. Writhing movements occur in the limbs, typically initially in the hands and feet; it can also involve the neck and trunk muscles.

Dysphagia Difficulty swallowing.

Dystonia A muscle spasm, often in the limbs or neck, which causes involuntary abnormal positioning, often with obvious over-activity of the muscles involved.

Electroconvulsive therapy/ECT (electroshock treatment). A treatment in psychiatry where electrical impulses are used for therapeutic effect. The main application in PD is for otherwise therapy-resistant depression.

Electron transport chain (respiratory chain). A series of protein complexes embedded in the mitochondrial membrane which transfer electrons through a sequence of oxidation/reduction reactions which generate energy within cells.

Excitatory flow Impulses transmitted along a nerve which result in increased activity.

Executive functioning Organization for day to day tasks, involving the frontal and prefrontal areas of the brain.

Fluid-attenuated inversion recovery (FLAIR) One of the sequences used in MRI scanning, used to remove the effects of fluid from the resultant images.

Free radical An atom, molecule, or ion with unpaired electrons which is, as a result, highly reactive and can cause damage to cell structure.

Frontal cortex The anterior surface of the brain, involved with reasoning, planning, and other complex cognitive functions.

G-protein Guanine nucleotide binding proteins. These are a family of cell-membrane proteins involved in second messenger pathways. One group stimulates the production of cyclic AMP while another inhibits it.

Glial cytoplasmic inclusions These are seen on histology of brains from patients with multiple system atrophy. They can be considered the equivalent in MSA of the Lewy bodies in PD brains.

Globus pallidus (Latin for 'pale globe'.) One of the basal ganglia, situated between the thalamus and the putamen. It is divided into two segments, internal (GPi) and external (GPe); the GPi is a common site for surgical lesioning or stimulation in the advanced PD patient.

Glutamate A widespread neurotransmitter with an excitatory function. Abnormal levels occur in several brain diseases including PD, which are associated with cell damage through abnormal entry of calcium into cells.

High-field MRI scanning An MRI system that operates at a higher magnetic field strength than conventional systems, to produce clearer, more detailed images.

Hydrocephalus Abnormal accumulation of cerebrospinal fluid in the cavities (ventricles) of the brain.

Hypomimia Reduced facial expression sometimes called a mask-like expression, typical of PD.

Hypophonia A reduction in vocal volume and modulation such that the patient has a monotonous voice.

Hypothalamus The area of the brain lying at the top of the brainstem, just below the thalamus. It regulates metabolic processes and other parts of the autonomic nervous system. The hypothalamus releases hormones which influence the pituitary gland.

Impulse control disorder A collective term for addictive behaviours such as pathological gambling, hypersexuality, and compulsive shopping.

Inhibitory flow Impulses transmitted along a nerve which result in reduced activity.

Intermediate reticular zone Located within the brainstem, an area of the medulla involved in automatic control of breathing, heart rate and blood pressure.

Kinesthetic (learning). A process of learning through physical activity rather than listening to a lecture or watching a demonstration.

Lacunar cerebrovascular disease Poor circulation or small areas of blocked circulation (strokes) occurring typically in the deeper or subcortical brain areas which can result in a form of PD known as vascular parkinsonism.

Levodopa/L-dopa Drug treatment for PD, available since the late 1960s. Levodopa is converted to dopamine in the brain and thereby functions as a replacement for deficient dopamine.

Lewy body A large inclusion within a nerve cell, composed of the protein alpha-synuclein. Lewy bodies are commonly found in the basal ganglia, but also in other brain areas such as the frontal cortex.

Lewy body dementia A condition of dementia where there is parkinsonism along with dementia and there are extensive Lewy bodies.

Lewy neurite A nerve cell containing abnormal proteins (including alpha-synuclein) and seen in patients with PD, dementia with Lewy bodies and MSA. The presence of Lewy neurites is closely related to the presence of Lewy bodies.

Ligand A marker or isotope which is typically injected and localizes to a body area and can be detected by SPECT scan or PET scan.

Livedo reticularis A discoloration in the limbs, typically the legs, which can occur as a reaction to drugs, e.g. amantadine.

Locus coeruleus (Latin for 'blue spot'.) A nucleus in the brainstem involved with the response to panic or stress. It contains melanin granules, hence the colouration of the area.

Medulla oblongata An area within the lower part of the brainstem which deals with automatic functions such as the control of breathing, heart rate, and blood pressure.

Micrographia Handwriting with a reduction in size and clarity.

Mid-commissural point An area in the middle of the flat layer of fibres that connect the left and right hemispheres of the brain (the commissural fibres). The mid-commissural point is half way between the front and back end of this layer, and is a reference point for deep brain surgery localization.

Midbrain Also known as the mesencephalon, an area in the brainstem including the lower end of the substantia nigra. It is situated just above the pons.

Mitochondrial complex Mitochondria are subcellular components that are responsible for energy production (*see also* electron transport chain). The pathways involved in this process are referred to as the mitochondrial complex.

Mitochondrial dysfunction Abnormality of the processes of energy production within cells as a result of damage within the mitochondria.

MMSE (Mini Mental State Examination). A 30-point scale used to score memory loss.

MPTP (1-methyl 4-phenyl 1,2,3,6-tetrahydropyridine). A chemical produced accidentally during illegal manufacture of recreational drugs, which causes a form of PD.

Muscarinic receptor One type of acetylcholine receptor which is the chemical opposite of the nicotinic receptor.

Myenteric plexus A neural network that regulates gut motility. These nerves also control the release of gastric juices during digestion. Degeneration of this plexus occurs in PD.

Myoclonus A sudden shock-like involuntary muscle movement. It can occur in the limbs, stomach muscles, and sometimes the entire body.

Neocortex The newest part of the cerebral cortex to evolve, the neocortex is arranged in six functionally distinct layers. It is involved in more advanced processes such as conscious thought, hearing, movement generation, and language.

Neuroleptic treatment (antipsychotic treatment). This drug treatment typically has some form of dopamine-blocking activity and can therefore result in a dopamine-deficiency syndrome including tremor and parkinsonism.

Neuromelanin The dark pigment in the brainstem and deep brain areas, such as the substantia nigra and the locus coeruleus, which stains black on brain slices and is a marker of the area which becomes affected in PD and similar disorders.

Neuroprotection The mechanisms or agents which protect nerve cells from degeneration and death. No treatment is currently considered neuroprotective for PD and current therapies are only effective in treating the symptoms.

Nigrostriatal pathway/nigrostriatal projections The nerve fibres connecting the substantia nigra with the striatum; this pathway degenerates in PD.

Nucleus basalis of Meynert One of the basal nuclei, which degenerates in dementia associated with PD.

Nystagmus Uncontrolled movement of the eyes occurring, for example, in patients with disease or degeneration of the balance centre or of the brainstem areas controlling eye movements.

Obsessive compulsive behaviour/disorder (OCD) A psychiatric condition in which obsessive thoughts, combined with anxiety, lead to repetitive tasks or rituals. One of the best known is compulsive hand washing, but numerous other types of behaviour can occur.

Oculogyric crisis An acute onset movement disorder in which there is involuntary upward deviation of the eyes and backward and lateral flexion of the neck. This is sometimes a side-effect of drugs, such as metoclopramide, and is more common in young females.

On/off effect of PD, occurring after a few years of treatment, in which the patient has a good response at times (the 'on' effect) but having a poor response at other times (the 'off' effect). Since the patient moves between these states, the fluctuation is referred to as an on/off effect (also known as motor fluctuations).

Orthostatic/postural hypotension A excessive fall in blood pressure and associated giddiness that occurs upon standing.

Osteomyelitis An infection of the bones or bone marrow.

Pallido-pyramidal degeneration A description of cell death occurring in the globus pallidus and also in the pyramidal tract, which is the routing of nerve fibres from the surface of the brain to the spinal cord.

Parkin A protein involved in a clearance system of other waste proteins and molecules (by-products or 'debris' from cell metabolism). Parkin is produced by a gene (the Parkin gene) which is mutated (i.e. abnormal) in a small proportion of patients with early-onset Parkinson's disease.

Parkinson-plus syndrome A collective term for conditions in which there is degenerative parkinsonism and additional involvement resulting from degeneration in other brain areas. Examples of Parkinson-plus are MSA and progressive supranuclear palsy. It is a descriptive term rather than a specific diagnosis, but can be useful when the features of a specific condition are not fully developed, and it is evident that the patient has more problems than would occur with PD alone.

Parkinsonism A combination of clinical features including bradykinesia and one or more of resting tremor, rigidity and postural instability. All patients with PD have parkinsonism, but not all patients with parkinsonism have PD (they could have drug-induced, vascular, or other types of parkinsonism).

Pericardial effusion An accumulation of fluid in the space between the heart and the pericardium (the lining that surrounds the heart). *See also* cardiac tamponade.

Perichondritis Inflammation of the membrane surrounding cartilage, particularly of the ear.

Positron emission tomography (PET) scan An image produced by the detection of positron emission from short-lived radioactive 'tracer' isotopes introduced into the body. Tissue uptake and relative blood flows (such as in brain activity) can be measured and mapped using computerized tomographic reconstruction to give a 3-D image. *See also* SPECT scan.

Placebo-controlled A clinical trial in which one half or a proportion of patients receive an inactive treatment (placebo) which appears identical to the active medication under test.

Pneumothorax Entry of air into the pleural cavity, which causes pressure on the lungs and results in breathing difficulties.

Pontine tegmentum An area within the brainstem where rapid eye movement (REM) sleep is controlled.

Post-encephalitic parkinsonism A form of parkinsonism that occurs secondary to encephalitis, a viral infection and inflammation of the brain. Resulting symptoms include fever, seizures, memory loss, speech difficulty, and loss of power. In the 1920s a worldwide epidemic of encephalitis broke out and many individuals subsequently developed parkinsonian symptoms.

Postsynaptic Neurones or nerve cells communicate with each other across a junction called a synapse. A chemical messenger (such as dopamine) is released from the presynaptic neurone, into the synapse (also called the synaptic cleft) and then taken up by receptors on the surface of the postsynaptic neurone.

Postural hypotension *See* orthostatic hypotension.

Praxis Forming purposeful movements and gestures. Abnormality of praxis results in dyspraxia or apraxia. Specific examples include inability to dress, hence dressing dyspraxia or apraxia.

Presynaptic *See* postsynaptic.

Psychomotor retardation Slowing down of thought and reduction of physical movements. This occurs in depression but is also seen in PD patients.

Punding Repetitive motor activity, often complex, such as repetitive reassembling of small electrical items, initially observed in patients abusing drugs like cocaine. Also more recently described in patients receiving certain dopaminergic therapy for PD.

Putamen One of the basal ganglia components which degenerates in PD. The putamen and caudate together form the striatum.

Raphe system A collection of nuclei which release serotonin, the neurotransmitter which is responsible for the control of mood. The Raphe nuclei are found in the medulla, pons and midbrain.

Retroperitoneal The peritoneum is the membrane that lines the abdominal cavity and contains most of the abdominal organs. The area behind this is the retroperitoneal area, where other organs, such as the kidneys, are located.

Serotonin Also called 5-hydroxytryptamine (5-HT). A neurotransmitter involved in mood; reduced levels have been linked to depression. Drug treatments can involve inhibiting the breakdown of serotonin, hence SSRIs (selective serotonin reuptake inhibitors). Serotonin has also been linked to the presence and severity of tremor in patients with PD.

Sialhorrhea Excess salivation.

Single photon emission computed tomography (SPECT) scan A 3-D image obtained by a gamma-ray camera that picks up signals from an injected isotope. SPECT scan machines vary from simple ones with one detector to those with several or multiple heads. *See also* PET scan.

Spinocerebellar syndrome A combination of problems occurring in the spinal cord and the balance centre of cerebellum, resulting in stiffness or spasticity in the limbs and poor balance.

Striatum The deep brain area responsible for controlling movement. The striatum is a collective term for the putamen and the caudate which are two of the key basal ganglia.

Substantia nigra Part of the basal ganglia, the substantia nigra appears as a black stain in section, due to the presence of neuromelanin. In Parkinson's disease the area degenerates, resulting in dopamine loss and loss of pigmentation. This is the primary area where PD degeneration is first seen.

Subthalamic nucleus One of the basal ganglia, situated below the thalamus. It is a target area for lesions or stimulation in deep brain stimulation of advanced PD.

Sundowning The onset or worsening of disorientation or confusion during the evening or night with improvement or disappearance during the day. Typical of dementing disorders such as PD or Alzheimer's disease.

Supranuclear gaze palsy A disorder (muscle paralysis) of eye movement resulting from damage in the area of the brainstem lying above the nuclei that connect the nerves to the eye muscles.

Sympathetic nervous system A component of the autonomic nervous system which is activated during stress, resulting in an increase in heart rate and blood pressure. Activation will also increase sweating, reduce gut motility, and give rise to dilation of the pupils and change in the hair follicles, resulting in them standing on end (pyloerection or goosebumps).

Thalamus One of the deep brain areas, which functions as a relay station for sensory and motor information.

Transcranial magnetic stimulation Brain stimulation by the passage of weak electric currents in magnetic fields. It has been conducted in mainly small-scale studies of PD and other neurological disorders like migraine and depression.

Tremor Rhythmic movement or oscillation which can affect the limbs, the head, and individual body parts such as the chin or tongue. 'Internal tremor' sensations are felt by the patient but are not visible to an observer.

Tremor-dominant A category of PD where tremor is a significant part of the clinical picture alongside less severe rigidity and bradykinesia.

Ubiquitin A small protein found in most complex cells, ubiquitin is part of a regulatory system (ubiquitin proteasome system) for removing degraded proteins from cells.

UPDRS score A universally recognized scoring system (Unified Parkinson's Disease Rating Scale) that measures the severity of PD.

Wearing off The symptoms that occur when Parkinson medication stops working. Typically, the patient will have a response to medication and a lessening of symptoms, but the benefit wears off before the next dose is due to be taken.

Index

Abbreviations

AA	atypical antipsychotic
AAC	augmentative–alternative communication
AChE	acetylcholinesterase
AD	autosomal dominant
ADAS-cog	Alzheimer's Disease Assessment Scale–cognitive portion
ADLs	activites of daily living
AIMS	Abnormal Involuntary Movement Scale
ANC	absolute neutrophil count
APDA	American Parkinson's Disease Association
AR	autosomal recessive
BDI	Beck Depression Inventory
Beta-CIT	[123I]ß-carbomethoxy-3-ß-(4-iodophenyl)-tropane (CIT)
BPRS	The Brief Psychiatric Rating Scale
CBC	complete blood count
ChAT	choline acetyltransferase
CI	confidence interval
CIBIC	Clinician's Interview Based Impression of Change
CNS	central nervous system
COMT	catechol-O-methyl transferase
CoQ10	coenzyme Q10
CR	controlled-release
CT	computed tomography
DA	dopamine agonists
DaTSCAN	dopamine transporter scanning (trade name for FP-CIT)
DBS	deep brain stimulation
DHEA	dehydroepiandrosterone
DLB	Dementia with Lewy bodies
DRS	Dementia Rating Scale
DSM	Diagnostic and Statistical Manual
ECT	electroconvulsive therapy
EDS	excessive daytime sleepiness
EDTA	ethylenediamine tetra-acetic acid
EECP	enhanced external counter-pulsation
ESR	erythrocyte sedimentation rate
ESS	Epworth Sleepiness Scale
ET	essential tremor
FDA	Food and Drug Administration
FDG-PET	flurodeoxyglucose positron emission tomography
FLAIR	fluid-attenuated inversion recovery
FLASQ-PD	Florida Surgical Questionnaire for PD
FP-CIT	fluropropyl-2,-carbo-methoxy-3,-(4-iodophenyl) nortropane
GABA	gamma-aminobutyric acid
GAD	generalized anxiety disorder
GCIs	glial cytoplasmic inclusions
GDS	Geriatric Depression Scale
GI	gastrointestinal
GPe	globus pallidus externa
GPi	globus pallidus interna
GSH	glutathione
HAM-D	Hamilton Rating Scale for Depression
HFD	high-frequency discharges
HY	Hoehn and Yahr
IADLs	instrumental activities of daily living
IBF	iodobenzofuran
IBZM	iodobenzamide
L-DOPS	L-threo-3, 4-dihydroxy-phenylserine
LRRK2	leucine-rich, repeat kinase 2
LSVT	Lee Silverman Voice Therapy
MAOB-I	monoamine oxidase B inhibitor
MIBG	meta-iodobenzylguanidine
MMSE	Mini Mental State Examination
MPP+	N-methyl-4-phenylpyridine
MPTP	1-methyl-4-phenyl-1,2,3,6-tetrahydropyridine
MRI	magnetic resonance imaging
MSA	multiple system atrophy
MSA-C	multiple system atrophy (cerebellar)
MSA-P	multiple system atrophy (parkinsonism)
MSLT	Multiple Sleep Latency Test
NE	norepinephrine
NMDA	N-methyl D-aspartate
NP	nurse practitioner
NPI	Neuropsychiatric Inventory
OCD	obsessive compulsive disorder
OSA	obstructive sleep apnoea
OT	occupational therapist
PA	physician assistant
PD	Parkinson's disease
PDD	Parkinson's disease with dementia
PDQ	Parkinson's Disease Questionnaire
PDSI	Parkinson's Disease Summary Index
PDSS	Parkinson's Disease Sleep Scale
PET	positron emission tomography
PLMS	periodic leg movements of sleep
PPRS	Parkinson Psychosis Rating Scale
PSP	progressive supranuclear palsy
PT	physical therapist
qhs	night-time dose
RBD	REM sleep behaviour disorder
REM	rapid eye movement
RLS	restless legs syndrome
SGOT/AST	serum glutamic-oxaloacetic transaminase
SGPT/ALT	serum glutamic-pyruvic transaminase
SNr	substantia nigra pars reticulata
SPECT	single photon emission computed tomography
SS	serotonin syndrome
SSRI	selective serotonin reuptake inhibitor
STN	subthalamic nucleus
TCA	tricyclic antidepressants
UK-PDRG	United Kingdom Parkinson's disease research group
UPDRS	Unified Parkinson's Disease Rating Scale
UPSIT	University of Pennsylvania Smell Identification Test
WBC	white blood cell
5-HT	5-hydroxytryptamine or serotonin